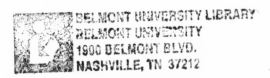

HUMAN EMBRYOLOGY

M.J.T. FITZGERALD & M. FITZGERALD

Human Embryology

Human Embryology

M.J.T. FitzGerald MD PhD DSc MRIA

Professor and Chairman, Department of Anatomy, University College, Galway, Ireland

and

Maeve FitzGerald MB BCh BSc

Senior Lecturer, Department of Anatomy, University College, Galway, Ireland

Baillière Tindall

LONDON   PHILADELPHIA   TORONTO   SYDNEY   TOKYO

This book is printed on acid-free paper

Baillière Tindall
W. B. Saunders

24–28 Oval Road
London, NW1 7DX

The Curtis Center
Independence Square West
Philadelphia, PA 19106-3399, USA

55 Horner Avenue
Toronto, Ontario, M8Z 4X6, Canada

Harcourt Brace & Company (Australia) Pty Ltd
30–52 Smidmore Street
Marrickville,
NSW 2204, Australia

Harcourt Brace & Company Japan
Ichibancho Central Building, 22-1 Ichibancho
Chiyoda-ku, Tokyo 102, Japan

Typeset by Create Publishing Services Ltd, Bath
Printed in Hong Kong by Dah Hua Printing Press Co Ltd

A catalogue record for this book is available from the British Library
ISBN 0-7020-1760-4

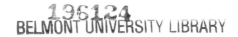

Contents

Preface

This textbook provides a clear, straightforward account of the sequence of events occurring between the moment of fertilization and the time of birth. It is designed for use by students of medicine and the allied health sciences, in conjunction with courses in gross anatomy.

All undergraduate embryology texts commence in the same general way, by following the course of development from fertilization to the point where, after some four weeks, the embryo has undergone a folding process and the elements of the principal body parts can be indentified. The remainder of development, up to the time of birth, is presented by systems (cardiovascular, digestive, etc.) in some texts and by region (thorax, abdomen, etc.) in others.

The regional choice has been taken for the present book. This is a logical choice because the various systems develop more or less simultaneously. The tissues and organs interact with one another as development proceeds, and the regional approach makes it relatively easy to describe and depict these interactions. A Systems Index is, however, provided on p. xi for students involved in courses where the approach is systems-based. The index will enable readers to make appropriate selections from relevant chapters.

Acknowledgements

Most of the photographs for this book were taken at the Carnegie Institution of Embryology, Washington DC, the Department of Anatomy, Cambridge University, and the Department of Pediatrics, University of Washington, Seattle. We wish to express our gratitude to the authorities concerned. Dr S. Viragh, Professor of Pathology at the Postgraduate Medical University, Budapest, kindly provided scanning electron micrographs of the embryonic heart and face. For his authoritative opinions on drafts of chapters dealing with the cardio-vascular system, we are greatly indebted to Dr R. H. Anderson, Professor in Pediatric Cardiac Morphology at the National Heart and Lung Institute, London.

We are pleased to acknowledge the advice and support of our publishing colleagues at Baillière Tindall, and the expertise and patience of Gillian Lee Illustrators.

Systems Index

General Embryology

1

Basic concepts

Human embryology is the science concerned with human development in the prenatal period. The prenatal period of life commences at the moment of fertilization, and terminates at birth.

WHY STUDY EMBRYOLOGY?

There are two good reasons why students of medicine and allied health sciences need to study embryology:

- It sheds light on the gross (topographic) anatomy of the body, because the gross anatomy is the endpoint of the process of development.
- It helps to explain the anatomy of congenital malformations.

ABOUT THIS BOOK

The book differs from other current embryology texts in being organized for the most part on a regional basis, rather than by systems. The underlying purpose is to allow the subject to be learned in conjunction with any ongoing course in gross (topographic) anatomy. Following mastery of the general features of development (Chapters 1–9), regional development can be followed in any order of choice, in step with the gross anatomy program.

A bonus of the regional approach is that the simultaneous study of different systems, within a given region, permits an immediate appreciation of the way in which they impinge on one another as they develop.

Embryology has its own vocabulary. As reading proceeds, it is important that embryological terms be clearly understood. They are introduced in *italics*, and are listed at the end of the chapters in which they are introduced. A Glossary of Embryological Terms is also provided at the end of the book. Terms specific to gross anatomy are in **bold** print in the text.

SOME EMBRYOLOGICAL TERMS

The term *fertilization* refers to the union of the spermatozoon with the oocyte, which usually takes place near the outer end of the oviduct within a few hours after ovulation. The term *conceptus* refers to the products of fertilization. The conceptus comprises the embryo, together with supporting tissues called *adnexa*, or *membranes*. The principal adnexa are the placenta and the amniotic membrane.

The exact date of fertilization is not usually known, because the event cannot be detected. It is customary, instead, to calculate the age of the conceptus from the first day of the last menstrual period. This is known as the *menstrual* or *gestational age*. It is

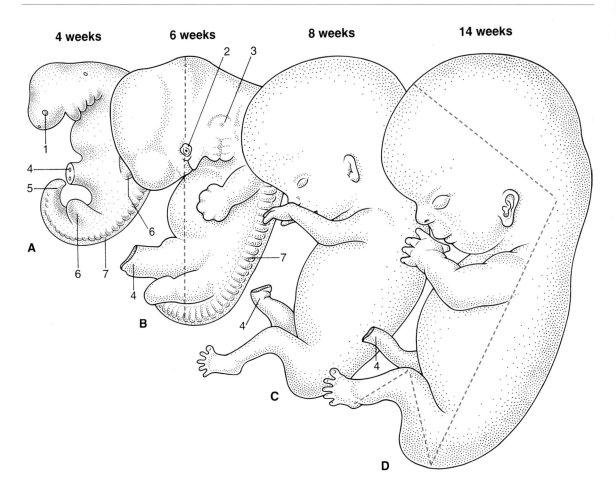

Figure 1.1. Three embryos and one fetus. The red dashed line in B is sitting height; in D, is standing height. 1, lens placode; 2, eye; 3, auricle (pinna); 4, umbilical cord; 5, tail; 6, limb bud; 7, somites.

about 2 weeks longer than the *postovulatory* or *fertilization age*, because the oocyte is usually fertilized 2 weeks after the preceding menstruation commenced.

Implantation is the process whereby the conceptus embeds itself in the mucous membrane (endometrium) of the uterus.

The *preimplantation period* of development is the interval, about 6 days in length, between fertilization and implantation. The *embryonic period* extends from commencement of implantation until the end of the 8th week after fertilization. The *fetal period* is from the beginning of the 9th week until the

moment of birth.

Embryologists describe the state of development of embryos by *stages* rather than by chronological age. This is because of the variable length of time that it takes for the conceptus to pass the numerous milestones of development. The 4-week-old embryo shown in *Figure 1.1A*, for example, is reckoned to be at Stage 13 because the lens placode (forerunner of the lens of the eye) is in place, and the lower limb buds have just appeared. This level of development may be attained as early as day 27 or as late as day 29. The 6-week embryo in *Figure 1.1B* shows features characteristic of Stage 17; this level of development may be attained between day 40 and day 44.

Embryonic stages will not be referred to further in this book. Enough has been said to indicate that the chronological dates given with most of the illustrations are approximate, rather than exact.

The two embryos mentioned above exhibit serially arranged clumps of embryonic connective tissue, called *somites*. Somites are a characteristic feature of segmented vertebrates. Their products include the vertebral column, as well as the segmentally innervated musculature of the trunk. The *somite period* of development extends from day 20 to day 30. The somites make their appearance during this time. They are still visible at 6 weeks (*Figure 1.1B*). By 8 weeks (*Figure 1.1C*) they have undergone differentiation (see below).

The size of embryos is expressed in the form of the *sitting height* (*crown–rump length*), which is measured from the crown of the head to the convexity of the rump (*Figure 1.1B*). The s*tanding height* tends to be used for fetuses; this includes the lower limb down to the heel (*Figure 1.1D*).

By the end of the embryonic period (*Figure 1.1C*), the greatest length of the embryo is some 30 mm – about equal to the top segment of the adult thumb. *Differentiation* – the development of distinctive cell types – is well under way. All of the major body systems have already been laid down. A brisk circulation is being maintained by a heart beating 160 times per minute, and the neuromuscular system is sufficiently differentiated to permit small movements of the trunk and limbs. During the fetal period, the main changes relate to growth rather than new developments. The single great exception is the brain, which continues to differentiate during the fetal period and infancy.

CONGENITAL MALFORMATIONS (ANOMALIES)

Congenital malformations are abnormalities of development that are present at birth. They occur in about 6% of live births. Half of them are detectable at birth; almost all of the other half become apparent during the first postnatal year.

The term *anomaly* is used in more than one sense. A *major anomaly* is a major congenital malformation, and a *minor anomaly* is a minor or trivial one. A long list of *inborn errors of metabolism* is included under the general heading of *congenital anomalies*. (Example: *phenylketonuria* (PKU), an autosomal recessive disorder resulting from phenylalanine hydroxylase enzyme deficiency.)

The definition of congenital malformations, given above, refers to live births. It should not obscure the fact that at least half of all conceptuses are malformed. In most cases the mother is unaware, because the conceptus fails to implant and is shed with the next menstrual flow. One pregnancy in five ends in *spontaneous abortion (miscarriage)* during the embryonic period. About one-third of spontaneous abortions result from deficient hormonal support from the corpus luteum within the ovary, for the implantation process. Another one-third are associated with abnormal development of the placenta. A final one-third are associated with malformation of the embryo.

Etiology of Congenital Malformations

Chromosomal Factors

About 0.5% of live-born infants have chromosomal aberrations. The great majority of the aberrations take the form of *trisomy*, where one of the gametes contains an additional autosome, as a result of *nondisjunction* (failure to separate) of a pair of autosomes during the first maturation division. Trisomies are most frequently associated with chromosomes 16, 21 and 22. Trisomy 21 is associated with *Down's syndrome*.

Chromosomal aberrations are found in more than 50% of early spontaneously aborted embryos (embryos expelled after implantation and before the end of the 8th week of development).

Genetic Factors

About 10% of congenital malformations are attributable to *single gene mutation* (molecular change within a single gene). Such mutations occur randomly, and subseqently show a Mendelian pattern of inheritance. They include many cases of congenital heart disease and of cleft lip and/or cleft palate. Mendelian inheritance is also a feature of a large number of inborn errors of metabolism.

Environmental Factors

Environmental factors associated with congenital malformations include infections, drugs and radiation. All are included under the general heading of *teratogens*. Teratogens may have the following effects:

- They are usually fatal during the first 2½ weeks of development. This is the critical, *predifferentiation period*, devoted to formation of the three germ layers.
- They are liable to produce major malformations with survival if active at any time during the rest of the embryonic period. All of the major body systems are laid down before the end of the embryonic period, and histodifferentiation gets well under way.
- During the fetal period, susceptibility to teratogens is greatly reduced, with the

exception of the brain, where differentiation is continuing.
- Genetic and environmental factors tend to act in concert. A genetic fault may predispose toward malformation of a body part, but expression of the fault often requires the additive effect of a teratogenic agent.
- Teratogens have specific loci of action. Some interfere with nucleic acid synthesis (and therefore with mitosis), others interfere with cell migration, others again with synthesis of cell products.

Infections precipitating malformations are almost always viral in nature, because bacteria cannot enter the embryo without first setting up an inflammation of the placenta – and this is a rare event. Viruses pass through the placenta with ease. By far the best known, and most dangerous, is the virus of *rubella* (German measles). At least one-third of affected infants show one or more malformations if the mother is infected before the end of the embryonic period. Malformations induced by rubella include deafness from damage to the cochlea, blindness due to cataract (opacification of the lens), and major cardiac anomalies. The most effective way to control the rubella virus is to vaccinate all children in the population.

Drugs precipitating malformations include alcohol, antimitotic drugs used to treat cancer, some drugs used to suppress epileptic seizures, and others used to relieve depression or anxiety. A large number are suspected of being teratogenic, but are difficult to incriminate with certainty because of the baseline incidence of malformations even when no drugs are taken. Hence the advice to refrain from drugs of any kind during early pregnancy.

Radiation, in the form of X-rays and gamma rays, is notoriously teratogenic – especially to the brain and the eyes – if the embryo is directly exposed to large amounts.

However, the small doses used in diagnostic radiology are not significant, provided the pelvic region is not included in the procedure in early pregnancy.

EMBRYOLOGICAL TERMS

(*Italics* in all chapters refer to malformations.)

Conceptus. Adnexa/membranes. Menstrual/gestational age. Postovulation/fertilization age. Implantation. Preimplantation period. Embryonic period. Stages of embryonic development. Somites. Somite period. Greatest length/crown–rump length. Standing height. Differentiation. *Congenital malformation. Major/minor anomalies. Teratogenic agents. Nondisjunction of autosomes. Single gene mutation.*

2

Fertilization and cleavage

THE MATURE OVARIAN FOLLICLE

Figure 2.1A shows the ovary, oviduct (Fallopian tube), and uterus. Fertilization usually takes place in the ampulla, close to the outer end of the oviduct. Part of the ovary is enlarged in *Figure 2.1B*, which depicts a mature ovarian follicle on the point of rupture. Within the follicle, the *oocyte* is surrounded by the homogeneous *zona pellucida*. Cells of the *stratum granulosum* line the inside of the follicular wall and form the *cumulus oophorus* around the oocyte. Outside the stratum granulosum is the cellular *theca interna*, which secretes luteinizing hormone (LH). The *theca externa* is a fibromuscular shell enclosing the follicle.

Two days prior to ovulation, the oocyte is still a *primary oocyte*, containing the full, diploid chromosome count (22 pairs of autosomes and 1 pair of female (X) sex chromosomes). It has remained arrested at an early stage of the first meiotic division (first reduction division) since before birth. On the last day before ovulation, it responds to a surge in pituitary gonadotrophin secretion, as follows:

• The first meiotic division is completed (*Figure 2.2A,B*). The cell division is very unequal, nearly all of the cytoplasm being retained in one of the daughter cells, the *secondary oocyte*. The other daughter cell is the *first polar body*. Both cells contain a

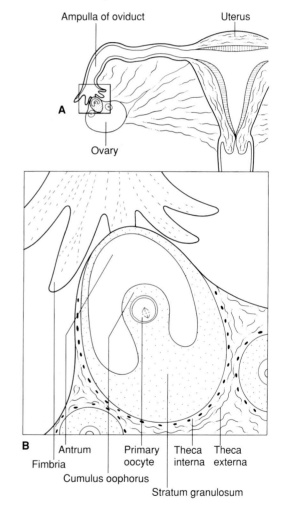

Figure 2.1. (A) Female genital tract. (B) Enlargement from (A) showing a mature ovarian follicle. The red ring represents the zona pellucida.

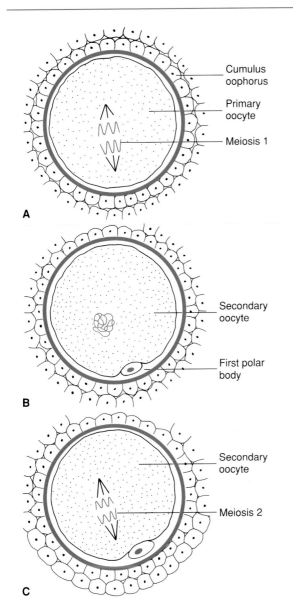

Figure 2.2. Events within the zona pellucida (red ring) prior to ovulation.

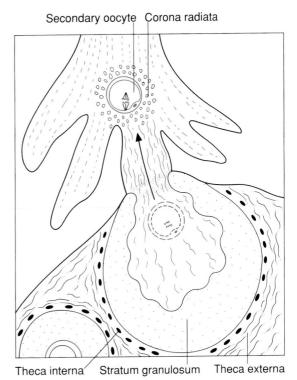

Figure 2.3. Ovulation.

OVULATION

haploid number of chromosomes, comprising 22 autosomes and one X chromosome.

- Without any DNA replication, the secondary oocyte enters a second meiotic division. This one proceeds as far as metaphase (*Figure 2.2C*). It will not progress further unless it is fertilized.

Prior to rupture, the ovarian follicle forms a blister at the surface of the ovary, as shown in *Figure 2.1*. Its cavity or *antrum* contains a large amount of follicular fluid. At the moment of ovulation, the follicle ruptures through the surface of the ovary. The liquor folliculi spills into the peritoneal cavity, along with the secondary oocyte surrounded by 2000–3000 cells of the cumulus oophorus. During the next few hours, the cumulus cells secrete a gelatinous extracellular ground substance. The cells and ground substance constitute the *corona radiata* (*Figure 2.3*).

The fimbriated end of the oviduct (Fallopian tube) is closely applied to the ovary at this time. One of the fimbria, the *ovarian fimbria*, exerts a sweeping action which moves the corona radiata–oocyte complex into the canal of the oviduct. The movement is assisted by the beating of cilia projecting from the lining epithelium. The oocyte remains viable (i.e. it can be fertilized) for up to 24 hours after ovulation.

Some women feel a sharp lower abdominal pain, known as *mittelschmerz* (*'middle pain'*, meaning mid-cycle pain) at the moment of ovulation. The pain is experienced on the same side as the affected ovary.

The granulosa cells remaining in the ovarian follicle enlarge and become tinged with yellow pigment called *lutein*. These *granulosa-lutein cells* secrete progesterone, which is primarily responsible for the post ovulatory build-up of the endometrium (the secretory phase of the menstrual cycle). At the same time, *theca-lutein cells* of the theca interna secrete estrogen, which is also involved in endometrial thickening.

If fertilization does not occur, the corpus luteum degenerates, and the loss of its hormonal output precipitates menstruation. On the other hand, if fertilization does occur, cells belonging to the conceptus called the *trophoblast* begin to secrete *human chorionic gonadotropin* (hCG) within a week. hCG causes the corpus luteum to persist, and to grow to nearly half the size of the ovary. This is the *corpus luteum of pregnancy*, and it persists for about three months. By the end of the third month, sufficient estrogen and progesterone are being produced by the trophoblast to sustain the pregnancy.

FERTILIZATION

A mature sperm cell (spermatozoon) comprises a head, neck, and tail (*Figure 2.4A*). A thin film of cytoplasm underlies the cell membrane.

Within the head is a highly condensed nucleus containing a haploid number of chromosomes – 22 autosomes and either an X or a Y sex chromosome. The leading half

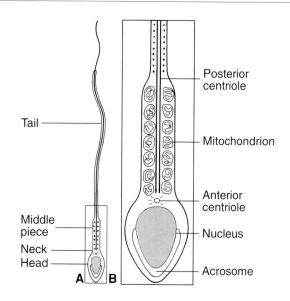

Figure 2.4. (A) Spermatozoon. (B) Enlargement from (A).

of the head is covered by the membrane-bound *acrosome*, derived from the Golgi apparatus (*Figure 2.4B*). The anterior centriole encircles the neck and the posterior centriole forms the tail or flagellum. The anterior part of the tail (the *middle piece*) is distinguished by a cuff of mitochondria providing energy for swimming movements.

During coitus, some 300 million sperms are contained in the 5 ml of semen deposited in the upper part of the vagina. Only about 1% enter the uterine cervix, the rest being lost by drainage from the vagina.

Around the time of ovulation, the mucous secretion of the cervix is less viscous than at other times. The 'thin' mucus is suited to the swimming action of the sperm tails. Rhythmic contractions of the uterus and oviduct assist passage of sperms; some reach the ampulla within ten hours of intercourse. The total number having an opportunity to fertilize the oocyte is about one hundred. Most survive for 24–48 hours, but a few may last for up to 4 days – a potentially significant period if intercourse has occurred within the week *before* ovulation.

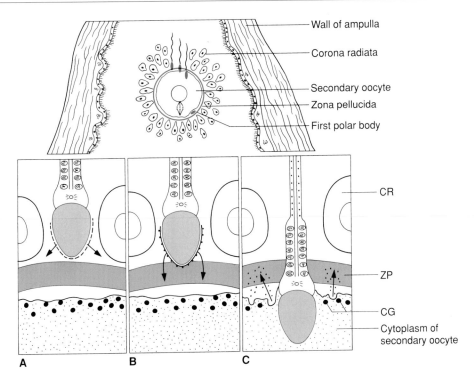

Figure 2.5. Diagrams of three steps in the fertilization process. A single sperm is represented three times. (A) Penetration of the corona radiata (CR); arrows indicate release of hyaluronidase enzyme. (B) Penetration of zona pellucida (ZP); arrows indicate release of acrosin. (C) Penetration of oocyte; arrows indicate release of cortical granules (CG) from the oocyte.

During their ascent through the uterus, the sperms become *capacitated*: a glycoprotein coating conferred on them during their stay in the epididymis is removed by proteolytic enzymes secreted by the uterine glands. Until the coat has been removed, sperms do not have the capacity to fertilize the oocyte.

Sperms close to the corona radiata show the *acrosome reaction* (*Figure 2.5A*). During the reaction, multiple points of fusion occur between the outer acrosomal membrane and the plasma membrane of the oocyte, permitting escape of acrosomal contents. Hyaluronidase enzyme released from the acrosome has a solvent action on the ground substance of the corona radiata, causing dispersal of the corona cells.

The first sperm to reach the zona pellucida binds to receptor molecules embedded in the surface of the zona. The receptor is thereby activated, causing release of an enzyme (acrosin) from the inner acrosomal membrane (*Figure 2.5B*). Acrosin facilitates penetration of the zona by the sperm head.

The first sperm to penetrate the zona pellucida exhibits fusion of the plasma membrane still covering the posterior part of the head of the sperm, with the plasma membrane of the oocyte (*Figure 2.5C*). The act of fusion induces exocytosis of *cortical granules* located just beneath the surface of the oocyte. The granules inactivate the sperm receptor molecules on the zona pellucida, preventing penetration of the zona by additional sperms.

The time taken for penetration of the corona radiata, zona pellucida and oocyte is less than 20 minutes.

The act of fusion triggers completion of

the second meiotic division of the oocyte. Like the first, the second meiotic division is highly unequal, one daughter cell receiving only a minute amount of cytoplasm before being jettisoned as the *second polar body* (*Figure 2.6A,B*). The other is the *definitive oocyte* – in lay terminology, the egg. Its nucleus contains 23 chromosomes (22 + X) and is called the *female pronucleus*.

The successful spermatozoon sheds the rest of its cell membrane while completing its penetration. The tail thrusts the sperm nucleus close to the female pronucleus before becoming detached. The nucleus swells and becomes the *male pronucleus*. The cell with its two pronuclei is the *zygote*.

The chromosomes of the two pronuclei replicate their strands of DNA, each forming 23 pairs of chromatids. The pronuclear membranes break down and the 46 chromosomes arrange themselves around the metaphase plate of the first mitotic division (*Figure 2.6C*).

Union of the female pronucleus (chromosomal constitution 22 + X) with a male pronucleus of constitution 22 + X will yield a female zygote (44 + XX, also written 46,XX). Union with a male pronucleus of constitution 22 + XY will yield a male zygote (44 + XY, also written 46,XY).

The zygote is about 0.15 mm in diameter. Although it is the largest cell in the body, it is scarcely visible to the naked eye. It is a seemingly simple cell with no dramatic ultrastructural features, but at the molecular level it is the most sophisticated of all biological systems. It multiplies prodigiously to yield the countless millions of cells that make up the tissues, organs and systems of postnatal anatomy – in a word, it is *totipotent*. Its genetic composition will determine that the individual will be not alone human, but unique – from the pattern of the fingerprints to the number, color, shape and length of the eyelashes.

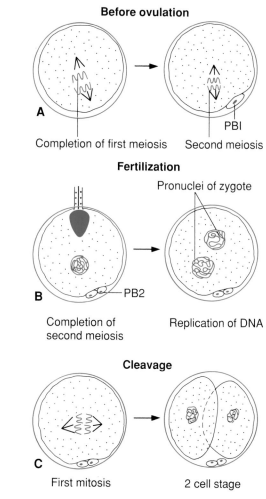

Figure 2.6. Summary of nuclear events in the oocyte.

CLEAVAGE

A *cleavage furrow* develops around the equator of the zygote, while the anaphase and telophase steps of mitosis are being completed (*Figure 2.7A*). Equal numbers of maternal and paternal chromosomes pass to each of the daughter cells. The daughter cells and their progeny are called *blastomeres*.

The cleavage process is repeated during the following 4 days, during which time the conceptus is wafted along the oviduct by ciliary action of the lining epithelium. There is active synthesis of fresh DNA by the blas-

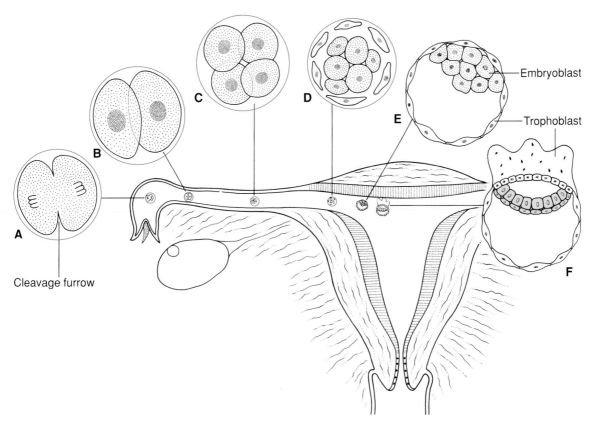

Figure 2.7. Events during the first 6 days of embryonic development. (A) Cleavage of zygote. (B), Two-cell embryo. (C) Four-cell embryo. (D) Morula. (E) Blastocyst. (F) Commencement of implantation. The transformation of the embryoblast in F is explained in Chapter 4.

tomeres in the interval between successive mitoses; however, fresh cytoplasm is not synthesized, and the overall size of the blastomeres diminishes progressively (*Figure 2.7B–D*).

The first three cleavages are almost synchronous. Later cleavages are asynchronous; the central cells divide less frequently and remain relatively large and round while the cells in contact with the inner aspect of the zona pellucida become flat (*Figure 2.7D*).

On the 4th day after fertilization the conceptus consists of 16–20 cells and is known as a *morula* (*Figure 2.7D*). On this day, as a rule, it enters the uterine cavity.

Within one day of arrival in the uterus, the zona pellucida is digested by uterine secretons, and fluid accumulates in the inter-

val between the peripheral and central cells of the morula. By the end of the 5th day, a *blastocyst* has been defined, comprising a shell of flattened cells, the *trophoblast*, and a central group of about 16 rounded cells, the *embryoblast* (*Figure 2.7E*). The trophoblast will form the placenta. The embryoblast will form the entire embryo.

Implantation of the blastocyst into the wall of the uterus commences on the 6th day after fertilization (*Figure 2.7F*).

ASSISTED REPRODUCTIVE TECHNOLOGIES

In vitro fertilization with embryo transfer (IVF-ET) is practiced in some 700 clinics throughout the world. The principal reason for using this kind of technique is inability of sperms to reach the ampulla of the oviduct following coitus. The usual cause is either obliteration of the canal of the oviduct by a previous infection, or diminished motility of the sperms.

The oviduct can be bypassed as follows: (a) Several follicles are induced to mature simultaneously, by systemic administration of gonadotropic hormones. (b) The oocytes are harvested, and cultured *in vitro* with capacitated sperms obtained from the male partner. (c) Fertilization and development are allowed to proceed for 3 or 4 days, whereupon the morula or blastocyst is placed in the uterine cavity, and allowed to implant in the normal way.

If the oviduct is patent, two other options are available. Following *in vitro* fertilization, the zygote can be introduced into the Fallopian tube (oviduct) ('zygote intrafallop-ian transfer,' ZIFT). Alternatively, aspirated oocytes can be mixed *in vitro* with capacitated sperms and immediately introduced into the tube ('gamete intrafallopian transfer,' GIFT). ('*In vitro*' translates as 'in glass' and denotes events occurring in test tubes or on slides.)

EMBRYOLOGICAL TERMS

Primary oocyte. Zona pellucida. Stratum granulosum. Cumulus oophorus. Theca interna. Theca externa. Secondary oocyte. First polar body. Follicular antrum. Corona radiata. Granulosa lutein cells. Theca lutein cells. Capacitation. Cortical reaction. Definitive oocyte. Second polar body. Female pronucleus. Male pronucleus. Cleavage furrow. Blastomeres. Morula. Blastocyst. Trophoblast. Embryoblast.

3

Implantation

On the 5th day after fertilization the zona pellucida is shed. The blastocyst enlarges by incorporating nutritive secretions ('uterine milk') exuded from the uterine glands.

On the 6th day, the blastocyst begins to implant in the endometrium (uterine mucous membrane). The endometrium is in the secretory phase of the menstrual cycle, which commences at the time of ovulation.

Three layers can be identified in the endometrium in the secretory phase (*Figure 3.1*):

- A *compact layer* comprising densely arranged stromal cells, the necks of uterine glands, and a capillary bed supplied by *spiral* endometrial arteries and drained by relatively straight endometrial veins. The spiral arteries are branches of the uterine

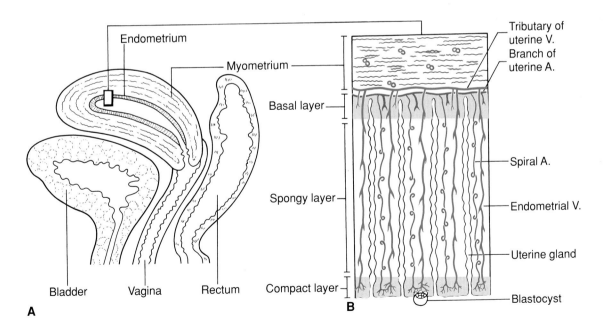

Figure 3.1. (A) Sagittal section of pelvic organs. (B) Enlargement taken from (A) at commencement of implantation. The blastocyst is enlarged in *Figure 3.2*.

artery which have penetrated the smooth muscle wall of the uterus (myometrium). The veins traverse the myometrium and drain into the uterine vein.

- A thick, *spongy layer* consisting of an edematous (swollen) stroma, the dilated bodies of uterine glands, and branches of the endometrial vessels.
- A *basal layer* containing the bases of the uterine glands. It has its own separate supply of basal blood vessels and it restores the integrity of the endometrium when the compact and spongy layers are shed, either during menstruation or during parturition (childbirth).

IMPLANTATION PROCESS

Implantation occurs most commonly on the posterior wall of the uterus. The surface of the blastocyst makes contact at a point overlying the embryoblast (*Figure 3.2A*). Upon contact, the trophoblastic epithelium becomes the cuboidal *cytotrophoblast* and engages in exuberant mitotic activity. The daughter cells shed their plasma membranes, creating a protoplasmic mass – the *syncytiotrophoblast* – filled with nuclei and organelles.

The syncytiotrophoblast secretes enzymes that attack the endometrium and hormones that help sustain the pregnancy. Enzymatic erosion of uterine glands liberates their contents for nourishment of the embryo. Nutrition is also provided by the stromal (connective tissue) cells, which become swollen with glycogen and lipid. The cytoplasmic changes in the stromal cells, known as the *decidual reaction*, commence at the implantation site and spread throughout the entire endometrium within a few days. *Decidual cells* are readily identified in superficial curettings (scrapings) of the endometrium and they are diagnostic of preg-

nancy. Following the decidual reaction the endometrium is henceforward called the *decidua*.

The mucous membrane of the cervix does not undergo any decidual change. It secretes a mucus plug that seals the cervical canal.

At the implantation site the capillaries of the compact layer are induced to sprout and to become dilated sinuses. Erosion of the sinuses results in spillage of maternal blood, creating a labyrinth of *lacunae* ('little lakes') within the syncytiotrophoblast (*Figure 3.2B,C*). Blood enters the lacunae from branches of the spiral arteries, and leaves by way of endometrial veins.

Human chorionic gonadotrophin (hCG) is a hormone secreted into the lacunae by the trophoblast. It reaches the ovary through the general circulatory system of the mother, and its function is to sustain the corpus luteum for the production of estrogen and progesterone. After the first trimester (three

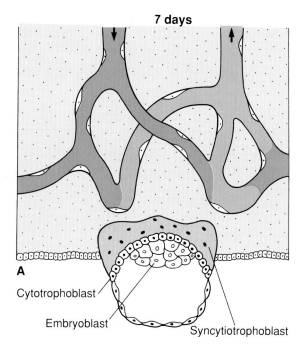

7 days

A

Cytotrophoblast

Embryoblast

Syncytiotrophoblast

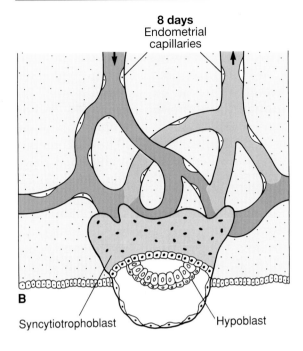

8 days
Endometrial capillaries

B

Syncytiotrophoblast · Hypoblast

months) of pregnancy the placenta produces these two hormones in sufficient quantity and the corpus luteum undergoes atrophy. hCG can be detected in the maternal blood and urine within a few days of the first missed menstrual period, *i.e.* about a week after implantation commences. Detection of hCG forms the basis of several pregnancy tests.

The conceptus is completely embedded by the 12th day after fertilization, and the breach in the overlying uterine epithelium has been repaired. The conceptus grows in the compact layer and in the outer part of the spongy layer, the deeper spongy layer being compressed.

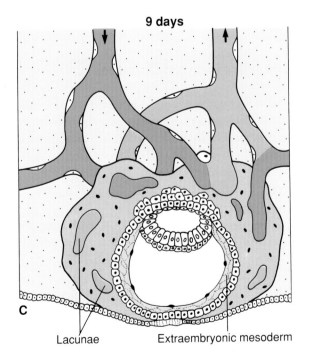

9 days

C

Lacunae · Extraembryonic mesoderm

Figure 3.2. The implanting conceptus on days 7–9 after fertilization. Arrows indicate direction of blood flow in endometrial capillary bed. (Uterine glands are not represented.)

Extraembryonic Mesoderm. Chorion

Originating from a layer of embryonic cells called the *hypoblast*, loosely arranged, branching cells occupy the cavity of the blastocyst (*Figure 3.2C*). These cells constitute the *extraembryonic mesoderm*. Where they line the internal surface of the trophoblast they constitute the *chorionic mesoderm* (*Figure 3.3A, p.18*). The mesoderm and trophoblast together constitute the *chorion*, and the fully implanted conceptus is known as a *chorionic vesicle* until the end of the embryonic period.

The extraembryonic mesoderm surrounding the embryo is linked to the chorion by a *connecting stalk* (*Figure 3.3B*). *Umbilical vessels* develop within the connecting stalk and link the chorionic vessels to others originating within the embryo itself.

14 days

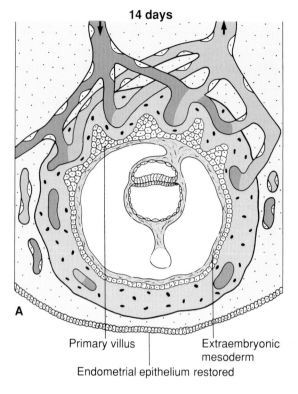

A

Primary villus

Extraembryonic
mesoderm

Endometrial epithelium restored

16 days

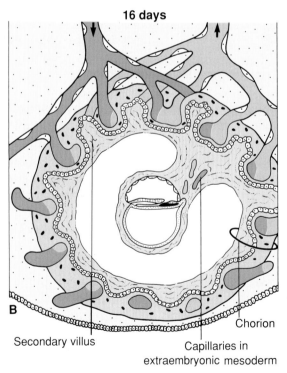

B

Chorion

Secondary villus

Capillaries in
extraembryonic mesoderm

Figure 3.3. Formation of chorionic vesicle.

Cytotrophoblastic Shell. Villi

Stems of cytotrophoblast divide in a T-shaped manner and link up with one another to create a *cytotrophoblastic shell* around the blastocyst (*Figure 3.4A*). The stems consist initially of trophoblast alone and are called *primary villi*. They become *secondary villi* when invaded by chorionic mesoderm, and *tertiary villi* when blood vessels develop within the chorionic mesoderm.

Secondary and tertiary villi are known as *chorionic villi*. They comprise *anchoring villi* attached to the trophoblastic shell, and *branch villi* that bud into the lacunae (*Figure 3.4B*).

Tertiary villi increase in number by repeated branching (*Figure 3.5A, p.20*). Embryonic and maternal blood are separated by villous capillary endothelium and trophoblast (*Figure 3.5B*).

Maternal and Embryonic Circulations

The *maternal circulation* comprises (a) the spiral arteries and their branches; (b) the intervillous space formed by the intercommunicating lacunae within the trophoblast; and (c) the endometrial veins. The *maternal blood* arrives in the uterine arteries and leaves in the uterine veins.

The *embryonic circulation* is anatomically separate from the maternal circulation. It comprises (a) umbilical arteries carrying blood from the embryo to the chorion; (b) the vessels of the chorionic villi; and (c) umbilical veins returning blood to the embryo. The embryonic blood cells are formed on the wall of the yolk sac.

Exchange of gases, nutrients and waste products between the maternal and embryonic blood streams commences early in the 4th week (see Chapter 7).

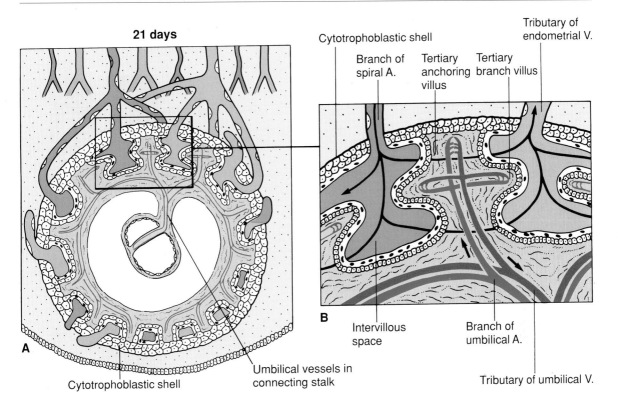

Figure 3.4. (A) Chorionic vesicle at 21 days. (B) Enlargement of upper part of (A) showing the circulation of embryonic and maternal blood. Red signifies oxygenated blood, blue, deoxygenated blood.

FORMATION OF THE PLACENTA

During the 3rd week, the chorionic vesicle begins to encroach upon the uterine cavity. The decidua at the original implantation site is called the *decidua basalis*, that enclosing the vesicle being the *decidua capsularis*. The *decidua parietalis* lines the remainder of the body of the uterus (*Figure 3.6A, p.21*).

After some 12 weeks of development, the decidua capsularis comes into contact with the decidua parietalis and begins to fuse with it (*Figure 3.6B*). In this way the uterine cavity is gradually obliterated.

Although the chorionic villi develop all around the blastocyst at first, they become progressively restricted to the decidua basalis. The *chorion laeve* ('smooth chorion') attached to the decidua capsularis eventually disappears. In contrast, the *chorion frondosum* ('leafy chorion') attached to the decidua basalis becomes an identifiable *placenta* by the end of the third month. The word 'placenta' means a cake, and refers to its discoid shape. The placenta is composed of a *chorionic plate* formed by the chorion frondosum, and a *basal plate* formed by the decidua basalis.

The structure and functions of the mature placenta are considered in Chapter 31.

IMMUNOLOGY OF PREGNANCY

Tissues transplanted from one region of an individual to another can survive and grow, because the *histocompatibility antigens* pres-

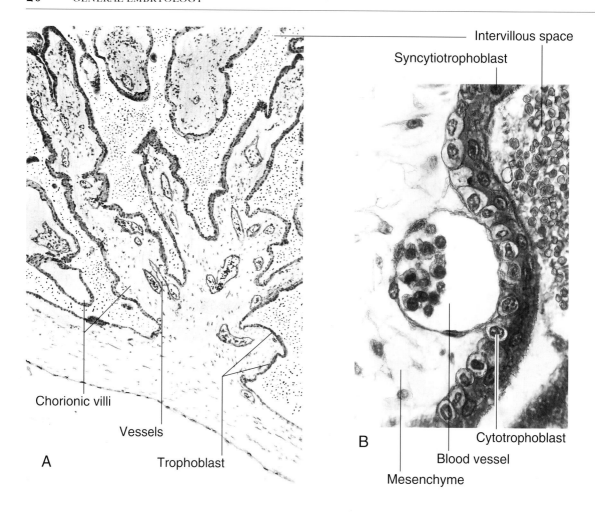

Figure 3.5. (A) Chorionic villi at 5 weeks. (B) Enlargement from adjacent section. (Cambridge Collection.)

ent in the membranes of the tissue cells belong to the same individual. On the other hand, tissues donated by one individual to another contain alien antigens which are detected by the immune system, leading to the production of antibodies and consequent tissue rejection.

Because half of the genetic material of the embryo is alien (from the father), some 'immunological filter' must be interposed between embryonic and maternal tissues. The most probable site of such a filter is the trophoblast. Trophoblastic tissue is relatively weakly antigenic, probably because it pro-

duces locally high levels of hCG, progesterone and corticosteroids.

PATHOLOGY OF EARLY PREGNANCY

Spontaneous Abortion

Spontaneous abortion (*miscarriage*), is the spontaneous termination of pregnancy before the end of the 20th week of pregnancy. It was pointed out in Chapter 1 that as many as 30% of conceptuses are so abnormal that they fail to progress beyond the

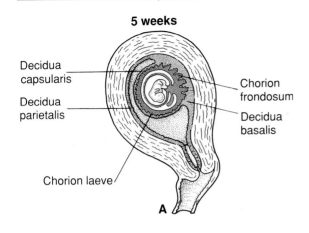

5 weeks

Decidua
capsularis

Decidua
parietalis

Chorion laeve

Chorion
frondosum

Decidua
basalis

A

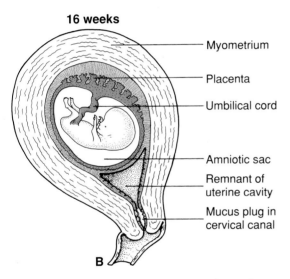

16 weeks

Myometrium

Placenta

Umbilical cord

Amniotic sac

Remnant of
uterine cavity

Mucus plug in
cervical canal

B

Figure 3.6. Diagrams illustrating changes accompanying enlargement of the chorionic vesicle.

blastocyst stage at best. These early abortions are not recognized as such because the conceptus is shed with a menstrual flow arriving on the due date.

In clinical practice, the commonest symptom of spontaneous abortion is that of delayed menstruation, where the blastocyst was not well embedded in the endometrium and is shed within a few days. Major malformations have been found in the great majority of such conceptuses, often including chromosomal abnormalities.

Causes of spontaneous abortion occurring later on include disease of the decidua, deficient function of the corpus luteum, viral infections such as rubella, and intake of drugs that are toxic to the embryo.

Ectopic Pregnancy

An ectopic pregnancy follows implantation of the blastocyst outside the uterine cavity. At least 95% of such implantations take place within the oviduct and last for 6–8 weeks. A classical presentation is that of a woman in her twenties who has had a previous lower abdominal operation for an infection such as appendicitis (with consequent development of scar tissue affecting patency of the oviduct). Amenorrhoea (absence of menstruation) is sustained for several weeks because trophoblast secretes hCG while eroding the wall of the tube. Sudden onset of lower abdominal pain signifies tubal rupture, and vaginal bleeding signifies detachment of the chorion frondosum, with leakage of blood into the uterine cavity.

Rarely, a blastocyst implants on the wall of the rectouterine pouch (of Douglas), having either failed to enter the tube or having been ejected from it. This is known as *primary abdominal pregnancy*. *Secondary abdominal pregnancy* is very rare, and follows rupture of a tubal pregnancy with secondary attachment of the trophoblast to a neighboring organ such as bladder or intestine. Abdominal pregnancies have been known to continue long enough for a viable fetus to be delivered by Cesarean section.

Trophoblastic Tumors

Hydatidiform mole is a benign trophoblastic tumor occurring in about 0.1% of pregnancies. The uterus becomes filled with swollen, grape-like villi which cause intermittent bleeding requiring complete evacuation of the uterus.

Choriocarcinoma is a highly malignant tumor which may develop from residual trophoblastic tissue retained in the uterus after evacuation of a mole. Initial symptoms of abdominal pain and vaginal bleeding may be followed by respiratory distress, indicating the occurrence of metastatic (secondary) tumor deposits in the lungs. Fortunately, these tumors are very sensitive to chemotherapy and survival is the rule unless the liver and brain have been invaded.

EMBRYOLOGICAL TERMS

Cytotrophoblast. Syncytiotrophoblast. Decidual reaction. Decidua. Lacunae. Extraembryonic mesoderm. Chorionic mesoderm. Chorion. Chorionic vesicle. Cytotrophoblastic shell. Primary, secondary, tertiary villi. Anchoring villi. Branch villi. Connecting stalk. Umbilical vessels. Intervillous space. Decidua basalis, capsularis, parietalis. Chorion laeve. Chorion frondosum. Placenta. Chorionic plate. Basal plate. *Spontaneous abortion (miscarriage). Ectopic pregnancy. Hydatidiform mole. Choriocarcinoma.*

4

The germ layers

EPIBLAST. HYPOBLAST

Early in the 2nd week after fertilization, the embryoblast resolves into two cell plates, the *epiblast* composed of tall columnar epithelium, and the *hypoblast* composed of low cuboidal epithelium. Together, they constitute the *bilaminar embryonic disc* (*Figure 4.1A,B*).

The margins of the epiblast give rise to a thin epithelial layer, the *amnion*, which together with the epiblast forms the *amniotic sac* (*Figure 4.1C*). As development proceeds, the amniotic sac expands enormously to surround the embryo and protect it from physical injury.

EXTRAEMBRYONIC MESODERM. PRIMARY YOLK SAC

From the margins of the hypoblast, branched cells invade the cavity of the blastocyst. These cells constitute the *extraembryonic mesoderm*. The innermost cells form a flattened epithelium (Heuser's membrane) enclosing a central cavity, the *primary yolk sac* (*Figure 4.1C*).

Spaces developing within the mesoderm coalesce to create the *extraembryonic coelom* (*Figures 4.1C* and *4.2*). The coelom splits the mesoderm into a visceral layer investing the amniotic sac and yolk sac, and a parietal layer which contributes to the chorion (Chapter 3). The visceral and parietal layers

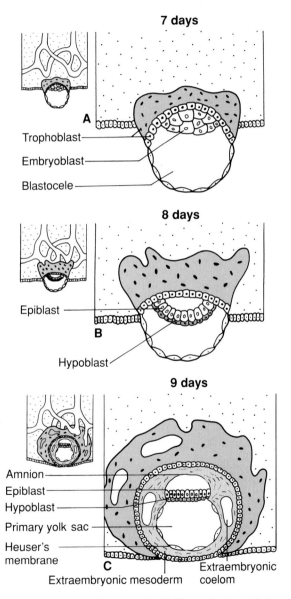

Figure 4.1. Early steps in differentiation of the blastocyst.

are linked by the *connecting stalk*, which is the forerunner of the umbilical cord (*Figure 4.2*).

PRECHORDAL PLATE. PRIMITIVE STREAK

Late in the 2nd week, the bilaminar embryonic disc becomes oval. The rostral part of the hypoblast thickens to form the *prechordal plate* (*Figure 4.2*). At the same time, part of the primary yolk sac is pinched off, and discarded into the extraembryonic coelom.

At the beginning of the 3rd week, the linear *primitive streak* makes its appearance in the caudal part of the epiblast (*Figure 4.3A,B*). The primitive streak is the site of very active cell migration. By a process of *invagination*, epiblastic cells dip through the streak and spread laterally beneath it (*Figure 4.3C*). Some of the migrant cells displace the underlying hypoblast and form the *embryonic endoderm*; the remainder form the *embryonic mesoderm*. Epiblastic cells that do *not* migrate remain as the *embryonic ectoderm*. These three

germ layers arise from the epiblast and they will form the entire embryo. The process of invagination resulting in the formation of the three germ layers is known as *gastrulation*.

The endoderm displaces the hypoblast completely by migrating inside the wall of the primary yolk sac (*Figure 4.4*). The endoderm-lined cavity is called the *secondary yolk sac*, or simply the *yolk sac*. A fingerlike projection, the *allantois*, extends from the yolk sac into the connecting stalk.

NOTOCHORD

At the rostral end of the primitive streak is a thickening, the *primitive node* (*Figure 4.5A*). A rod of cells grows rostrally from the primi-

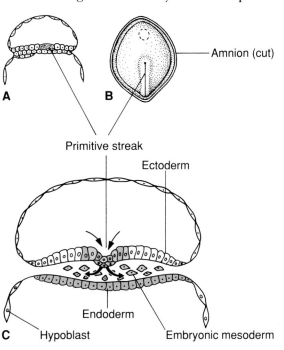

Figure 4.3. (A) Longitudinal section of embryonic disc. (B) Dorsal view of embryonic disc. (C) Transverse section at level of primitive streak. Arrows indicate directions of migration of epiblastic cells.

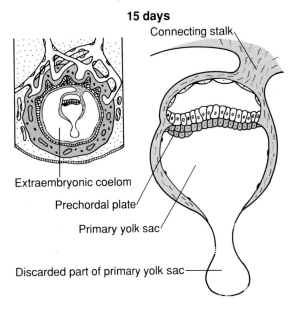

Figure 4.2. Prechordal plate; connecting stalk; reduction of primary yolk sac.

16 days

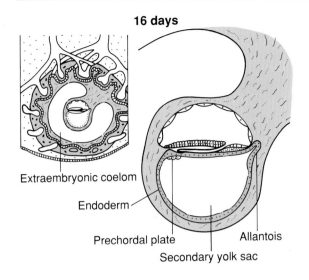

Extraembryonic coelom

Endoderm

Prechordal plate

Secondary yolk sac

Allantois

Figure 4.4. Longitudinal section of 16-day embryo.

tive node, beneath the ectoderm. This is the *notochordal process* and it reaches as far as the prechordal plate. Further extension is prevented by the adhesion of ectoderm to the prechordal plate, at the *oral membrane* (*Figure 4.5B,C*).

The notochordal process contains a canal extending from a pit within the primitive node. The floor of the notochordal canal and the underlying endoderm break down for a day or two, during which time the roof of the canal persists as the *notochordal plate*, and a *neurenteric canal* passes from the yolk sac into the amniotic sac (*Figure 4.5D*). Finally, the notochordal plate interacts with the endoderm before lifting out as the *notochord* proper (*Figures 4.5D* and *4.6*). The transformations preceding the appearance of the notochord proper are mainly of interest to comparative vertebrate embryologists.

THE TRILAMINAR EMBRYONIC DISC

Cells of the embryonic mesoderm migrate in three directions from the primitive streak (*Figure 4.5B–D*):

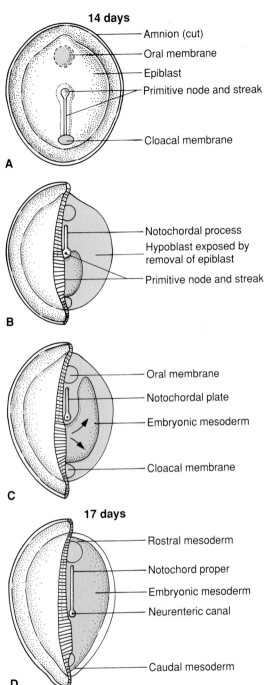

14 days

— Amnion (cut)
— Oral membrane
— Epiblast
— Primitive node and streak
— Cloacal membrane

A

— Notochordal process
— Hypoblast exposed by removal of epiblast
— Primitive node and streak

B

— Oral membrane
— Notochordal plate
— Embryonic mesoderm
— Cloacal membrane

C

17 days

— Rostral mesoderm
— Notochord proper
— Embryonic mesoderm
— Neurenteric canal
— Caudal mesoderm

D

Figure 4.5. Dorsal views of the embryonic disc. (A) represents the floor of the amniotic sac. In (B–D), the epiblast has been removed from the right side, to show migration of the embryonic mesoderm over the surface of the hypoblast.

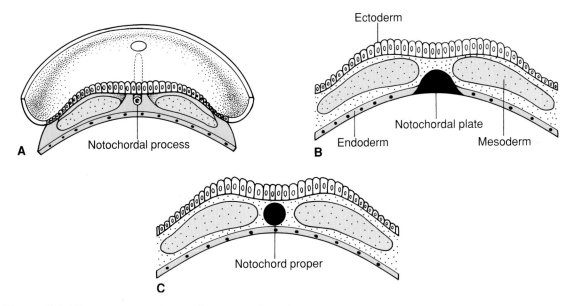

Figure 4.6. Transverse sections taken rostral to the primitive node, showing (A) the hollow notochordal process; (B) the notochordal plate fused with the endoderm; (C) the notochord proper.

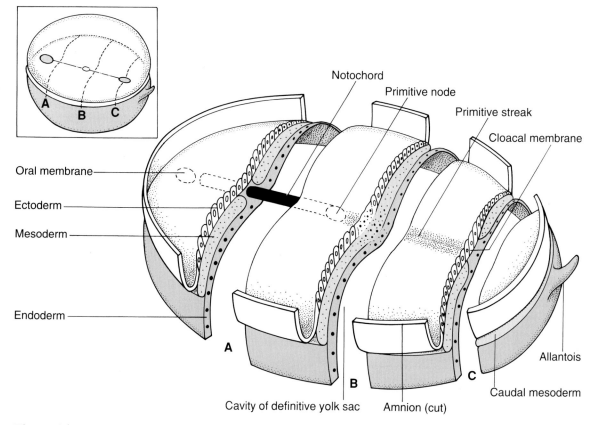

Figure 4.7. Stereosections of the trilaminar embryonic disc, viewed obliquely from above.

- Laterally, to the margins of the embryonic disc.
- Rostrally, alongside the notochord. The mesoderm skirts the oral membrane and blends across the midline at the rostral extremity of the embryo. In this book, the mesoderm rostral to the oral membrane is called the *rostral mesoderm*.
- Caudally, to skirt a second plaque of ectodermal–endodermal adhesion called the *cloacal membrane*. The mesoderm blends across the midline at the caudal extremity of the embryo. In this book, the mesoderm caudal to the cloacal membrane is called the *caudal mesoderm*.

The primitive streak continues to pay out mesoderm until the end of the 4th week. In its final days it retreats to the caudal extremity of the embryo. Very occasionally, persistent remains of the streak give rise to a tumor, called a *sacral teratoma*, containing tissues derived from more than one germ layer.

The oral membrane is the site of the future mouth. The cloacal membrane is the site of the future anal and urinary orifices (Latin, *cloaca*, 'sewer').

Mesodermal migration from the primitive streak converts the embryo into a *trilaminar embryonic disc* (*Figure 4.7*).

EMBRYOLOGICAL TERMS

Epiblast. Hypoblast. Bilaminar embryonic disc. Amnion. Amniotic sac. Extraembryonic mesoderm. Primary yolk sac. Extraembryonic coelom. Connecting stalk. Prechordal plate. Primitive streak. Invagination. Embryonic endoderm. Enbryonic mesoderm. Gastrulation. Secondary yolk sac. Yolk sac. Allantois. Notochord. Primitive node. Notochordal process. Notochordal plate. Neurenteric canal. Oral membrane. Rostral mesoderm. Cloacal membrane. Caudal mesoderm. *Sacral teratoma*. Trilaminar embryonic disc.

5

Initial differentiation of the germ layers

THE ECTODERM

Neurulation

The first signs of the nervous system appear when the notochord and paraxial mesoderm induce the overlying ectoderm to thicken in the form of a *neural plate* (*Figure 5.1A, B*). The cells forming the plate are called *neurectodermal cells*. The broader, rostral part of the neural plate is the *brain plate*. The narrower, caudal part gives rise to the spinal cord. The process of formation of the nervous system from the ectoderm is called *neurulation*.

On day 18 or 19, the neural plate shows a

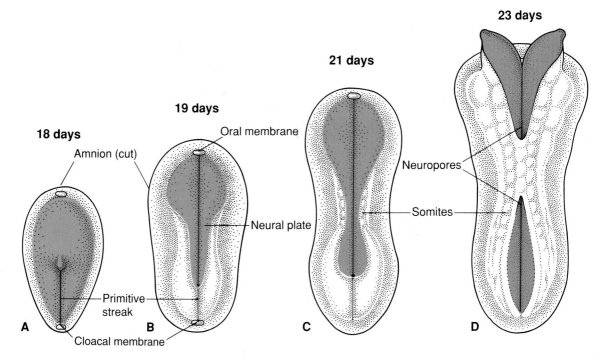

Figure 5.1. Dorsal views of the floor of the amniotic sac. The neural plate is shown in red.
Note: The somites and other parts of the mesoderm are seen through the surface ectoderm.

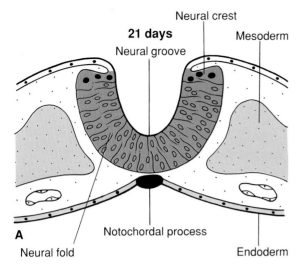

21 days

Neural crest

Neural groove

Mesoderm

Neural fold

Notochordal process

Endoderm

A

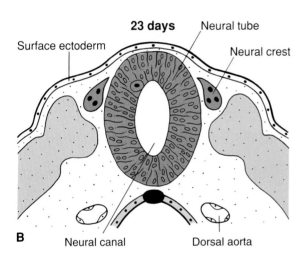

23 days   Neural tube

Surface ectoderm

Neural crest

Neural canal   Dorsal aorta

B

Figure 5.2. Transverse sections of the mid-region of embryos (C) and (D) in *Figure 5.1*.

midline *neural groove* flanked by *neural folds* (*Figure 5.1C* and *5.2A*). Early in the 4th week, the margins of the folds come together and form the *neural tube* (*Figure 5.1D* and *5.2B*). Fusion of the neural folds begins at the level of the fourth pair of somites, and proceeds simultaneously in rostral and caudal directions. Along the line of fusion a thin layer of mesoderm passes

between the tube and the restored *surface ectoderm*.

Cells close to the crests of the neural folds escape from the neural tube during closure. They lie alongside the neural tube, and constitute the *neural crest* (*Figure 5.2A, B*).

The ends of the neural tube are initially open, at the *rostral* and *caudal neuropores* (*Figure 5.1D*). The rostral neuropore closes off on day 25 or 26 and the caudal neuropore closes on day 27 or 28.

The neural tube forms the brain and spinal cord. The neural canal within the tube becomes the ventricular system of the brain and the central canal of the spinal cord.

Tissues Derived from the Ectoderm

Tissues derived from the *neurectoderm* include the central and peripheral nervous systems, the retina of the eye, and the posterior lobe of the pituitary gland.

Tissues derived from the *neural crest* include spinal and autonomic ganglia, the adrenal medulla and the pigmented cells of the skin and retina. Some neural crest cells arising from the brain plate behave like mesodermal cells, being capable of forming connective tissues.

Tissues derived from the *surface ectoderm* include the epidermis of the skin, together with hair follicles and cutaneous glands including the breast, the lens, the special sense cells of the inner ear, the anterior lobe of the pituitary gland, and the enamel of the teeth.

THE MESODERM

The Embryonic Coelom (Figure 5.3)

Late in the 2nd week, fluid-filled spaces appear within the rostral half of the embryonic mesoderm. The spaces coalesce during

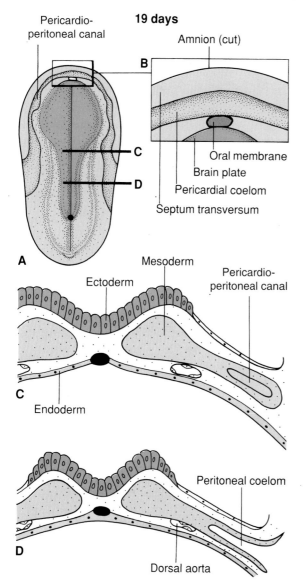

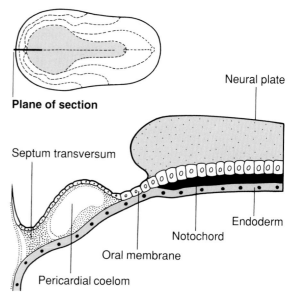

Figure 5.4. Median section of rostral end of 19-day embryo.

Figure 5.3. (A) Dorsal view of a 19-day embryonic disc. (B), Enlargement from the rostral part of (A). (C,D), Transverse sections at the levels indicated in (A).

the 3rd week, to create a U-shaped cavity, the *embryonic coelom*, which has three named parts:

- The rostral end of the cavity traverses the rostral mesoderm and is the *pericardial coelom (Figure 5.3A,B, and 5.4)*. The meso-

derm remaining at the rostral extremity of the embryo is called the *septum transversum*.
- The midregion on each side is the *pericardioperitoneal canal (Figure 5.3A,C)*.
- The caudal part, at mid-embryo level, is the *peritoneal coelom (Figure 5.3A,D)*. It displaces the investing film of extraembryonic mesoderm and opens into the extraembryonic coelom.

Subdivisions of the Embryonic Mesoderm (Figure 5.5)

Paraxial Mesoderm

The portion of the mesoderm nearest to the midline axis of the embryo is *paraxial*. For the most part, it undergoes *segmentation* in a rostrocaudal direction, creating the blocks of mesoderm called *somites*.

Days 20 – 30 constitute the *somite period*. During this period 34 or 35 somites are formed and are easily seen through the thin covering of surface ectoderm. They are more difficult to enumerate later on, but they continue to emerge until the end of the 5th week, with a total of 42–44 pairs. At appropriate levels they are called occipital, cervical, thoracic, lumbar, sacral or coccygeal.

The craniocaudal sequence of somite formation gives the rostral part of the embryo a 'head start.' By the time the most caudal somites are being defined during the 5th week, the most cranial ones have undergone 3 weeks of further development. Rostral regions of the mesoderm maintain their advantage throughout embryonic and fetal life. As will be seen when the circulation is considered in later chapters, the head, neck and upper limbs get the added boost of a preferential supply of oxygenated blood coming in from the placenta.

Intermediate and Lateral Mesoderm

The mesoderm lateral to the somites does not undergo segmentation. Next to the somites is the *intermediate mesoderm*. Outside this is the *lateral plate*, which encloses the pericardioperitoneal canal.

The part of the lateral plate beneath the surface ectoderm is the *somatic mesoderm*; 'soma' means 'body wall' in this context. The part next to the endoderm of the yolk sac is the *splanchnic mesoderm*, 'splanchnic' meaning 'visceral.'

Tissues Derived from the Mesoderm

The most cranial part of the paraxial mesoderm, rostral to the somites, fans out over the head and neck regions of the embryo as these develop. Tissues derived from it include part of the skull, and the muscles of the face and jaws.

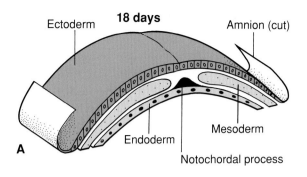

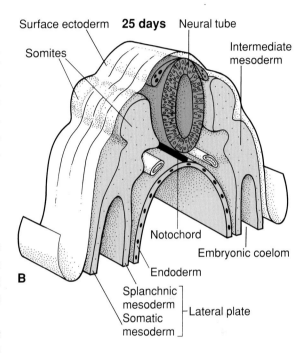

Figure 5.5. Early differentiation of the embryonic mesoderm.

- Tissues derived from the *somites* include the vertebral column and the skeletal musculature of the trunk; also the dermis (connective tissue of the skin).
- Tissues derived from the *intermediate mesoderm* include the kidneys and ureters, the gonads, the ductus deferens, and the uterus and uterine tubes.
- Tissues derived from the *somatic mesoderm* include the skeleton and musculature of

the limbs; also the sternum and the anterior parts of the ribs.

- Tissues derived from the *splanchnic mesoderm* include the cardiovascular system and the blood, the spleen, and the smooth muscle coat of the gastrointestinal tract.

THE ENDODERM

As will be shown in the next chapter, the dorsal part of the yolk sac becomes pinched off to form the embryonic *gut*. Tissues derived from the epithelium of the gut include the epithelia of the alimentary tract and of the glands opening into it (including liver and pancreas), and the epithelial lining of the lower respiratory tract and of the bladder and urethra.

EMBRYOLOGICAL TERMS

Neurulation. Neural plate. Brain plate. Neural folds. Neural groove. Neural tube. Neural crest. Rostral and caudal neuropores. Pericardial coelom. Septum transversum. Peritoneal coelom. Pericardioperitoneal canal. Paraxial mesoderm. Segmentation. Somites. Somite period. Intermediate mesoderm. Lateral mesoderm. Splanchnic mesoderm. Somatic mesoderm. Gut.

6

Folding of the embryo

Because of relatively rapid growth of the nervous system and mesodermal somites compared to that of the yolk sac, the trilaminar embryonic disc undergoes a process of *folding (flexion)* around its entire margin. Events in the longitudinal and transverse planes need to be described separately.

LONGITUDINAL FOLDING

The Phenomenon of Reversal

When the folding process is viewed in a progressive series of longitudinal sections, its profound anatomical significance can be appreciated. *Figure 6.1* contains three rather schematic sections to show the state of affairs at the beginning, middle and end of the process. Five structures have been numbered.

It is apparent that in *Figure 6.1A* the rostrocaudal sequence of the numbered items is entirely wrong with respect to their adult alignment. However, with the completion of the *head* and *tail folds* the sequence is entirely correct: the primordia of diaphragm and lower abdominal wall start out at opposite extremities of the embryonic disc and end up close to one another, as they should do.

Note in *Figure 6.1C* that the folding process imposes an hourglass constriction on the yolk sac, with partial extrusion of the sac from the embryo. The portion retained within the embryo is called the *gut*. The extruded portion is connected to the gut by the *vitelline duct*, which disappears later on.

Details of the Head and Tail Folds

Relationships at the conclusion of the flexion process are shown in *Figures 6.2* and *6.3*. The brain (with open rostral neuropore) overhangs the developing heart, which has invaginated into the pericardial coelom. The heart is ventral to the *foregut*, which is the compressed rostral end of the embryonic gut extending from the oral membrane to the opening of the vitelline duct. The septum transversum becomes wedged into the interval between the heart and the vitelline duct. Between the foregut and the brain, the notochord reaches rostrally as far as the oral membrane.

The *midgut* faces into the vitelline duct. The *hindgut* extends from the caudal margin of the vitello-intestinal communication to the cloacal membrane.

The caudal mesoderm has formed a fulcrum for the folding process, at the same time contributing mesoderm to the caudal part of the abdominal wall. The dwindling primitive streak has been carried onto the ventral surface of the embryo; it disappears before the end of the 4th week.

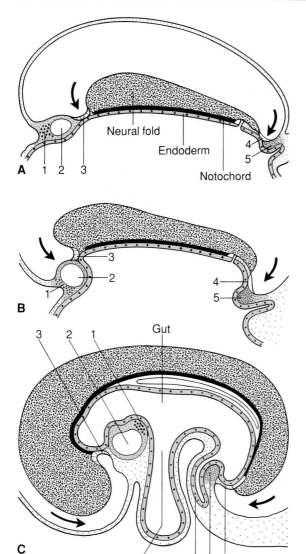

Figure 6.1. Scheme to illustrate the phenomenon of reversal. For the numbers, see text.

TRANSVERSE FOLDING *(Figure 6.4)*

The lateral margins of the embryonic disc give rise to the *lateral body folds*. The peritoneal coelom on each side initially opens outward into the extraembryonic coelom. Transverse folding causes the openings to be directed ventrally. Following constriction of the yolk sac, the openings communicate across the midline creating the **peritoneal cavity**.

Progression of transverse folding gives rise to the **umbilicus**, as shown in *Figure 6.5*. The rostral part of the umbilicus contains the vitelline duct and the caudal part contains the allantois. (The related blood vessels are described in Chapter 7.) Also present is a communication between the peritoneal cavity and the extraembryonic coelom. The opening is progressively reduced by ventral encroachment of the amniotic sac. The amnion comes to encircle and invest the vitelline duct and umbilical vessels, thereby defining the *umbilical cord*.

EMBRYOLOGICAL TERMS

Folding/flexion. Reversal. Head fold. Tail fold. Vitelline duct. Foregut. Midgut. Hindgut. Lateral body folds. Extraembryonic coelom. Umbilical cord.

Number in *Figure 6.1*	Embryonic structure	Relevant contribution to topographical anatomy
1	Rostral mesoderm	Part of diaphragm
2	Pericardial coelom	Pericardial cavity
3	Oral membrane	Marks site of future mouth
4	Cloacal membrane	Marks site of future anus
5	Caudal mesoderm	Infraumbilical abdominal wall

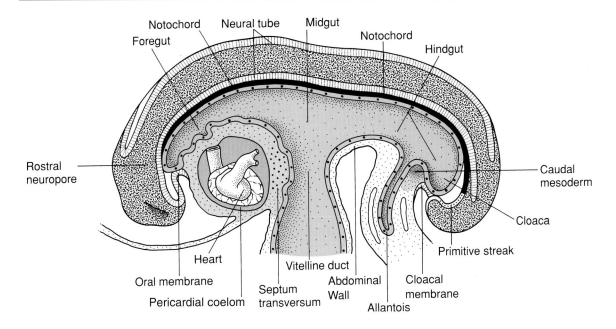

Figure 6.2. Longitudinal section of a 25-day embryo.

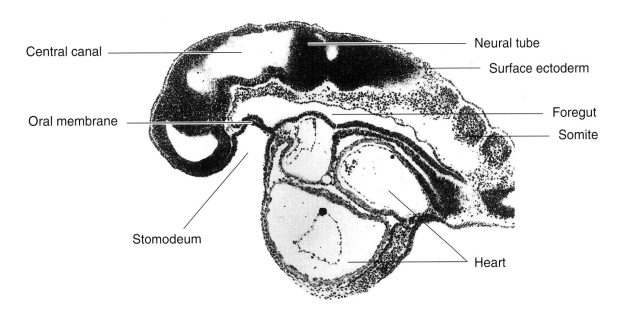

Figure 6.3. Longitudinal section of a 25-day embryo. The section is a little oblique, passing through neural tube rostrally and somites caudally. (Carnegie Collection)

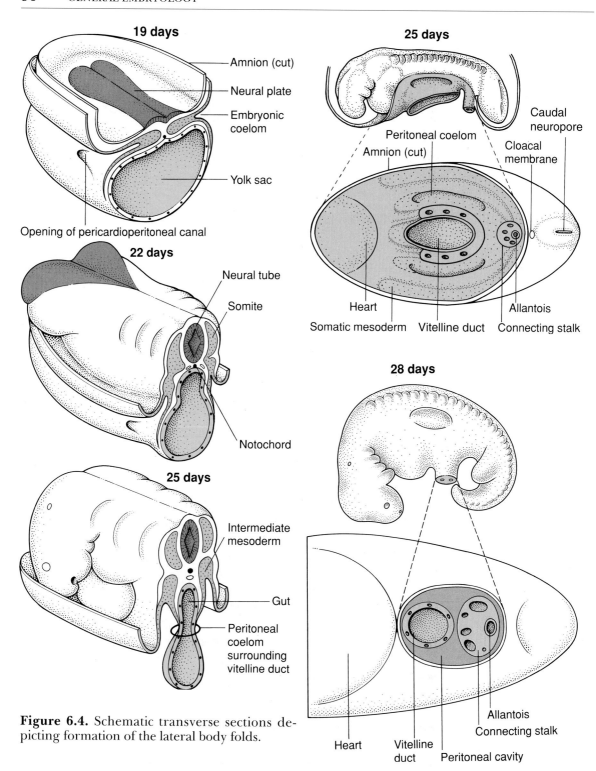

Figure 6.4. Schematic transverse sections depicting formation of the lateral body folds.

Figure 6.5. Development of the umbilicus.

7

Early cardiovascular system

By the end of the 3rd week of development, the embryo has become too large to be nourished by diffusion of nutrients from the yolk sac. For this reason, the cardiovascular system makes an early appearance, and an embryonic circulation begins to function early in the 4th week.

The developing heart drives three circulatory systems. One system collects red blood cells from the wall of the yolk sac and returns there for more; one collects oxygen and nutrients from the placenta and returns there with waste products; and one is contained entirely within the embryo in order to nourish it.

DEVELOPMENT OF THE BLOOD AND EARLY BLOOD VESSELS

Early in the 3rd week, *blood islands* appear in the extraembryonic mesoderm clothing the yolk sac (*Figure 7.1*). The central cells of each island are *hemocytoblasts*: they acquire hemoglobin and become primitive, nucleated red cells. The peripheral cells are *angioblasts* that form a capillary endothelium around each of the blood islands. Angioblasts also differentiate from the extraembryonic mesoderm of the connecting stalk and chorion. The endothelial chan-

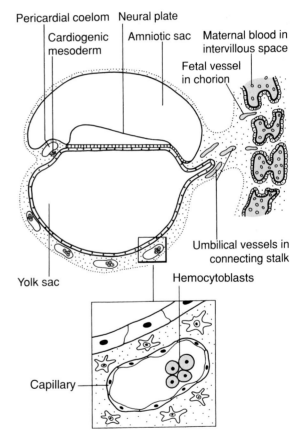

Figure 7.1. Longitudinal section of 18-day embryo, showing primitive vasculature.

nels extend into the embryo proper and link up with similar vessels developing within the embryonic mesoderm.

THE HEART TUBE

Prior to formation to the head fold, *cardiogenic mesoderm* occupies the floor of the pericardial coelom (*Figure 7.1*). A pair of *primitive heart tubes* develops from this part of the splanchnic mesoderm (*Figure 7.2*). When the folding process gets under way, they unite as a single heart tube. The tube sinks into the pericardial coelom, which is then called the *pericardial sac*.

Within the pericardial sac the heart tube buckles, assuming the shape of a twisted U (*Figure 7.3*). It gives rise to four *primitive heart chambers*, of which the *sinus venosus* is the most caudal.

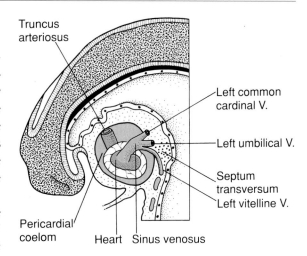

Figure 7.3. Primitive heart on day 25, showing inflow and outflow channels.

ARTERIES

Angioblasts developing within the paraxial mesoderm form a *dorsal aorta* on each side (*Figure 7.2*). The *truncus arteriosus* extends rostrally from the heart tube and is linked to the dorsal aortas by pairs of *aortic arches* differentiated from head mesenchyme. At the other end of the embryo, a pair of *umbilical arteries* develops in the connecting stalk and

links the dorsal aortas to capillaries within the chorionic villi. This completes the arterial component of the placental circulation.

Numerous *vitelline arteries* arise from the dorsal aortas and link up with the rich capillary bed on the surface of the yolk sac. The number of vitelline arteries becomes reduced to three that supply the gastrointestinal tract.

Finally, *intersegmental arteries* pass between successive mesodermal somites to supply the somites and the neural tube (*Figure 7.4*).

VEINS

Initially, numerous vessels carry red cells from the blood islands of the yolk sac to the caudal end of the heart tube. The larger ones resolve into a pair of *vitelline veins* which pierce the septum transversum to enter the sinus venosus (*Figure 7.3*).

Two *umbilical veins* develop in the connecting stalk (*Figure 7.1*). They link up with capillaries in the chorionic villi, and they bud rostrally within the somatic part of the lateral plate mesoderm to reach the heart (*Figures 7.4–7.6*).

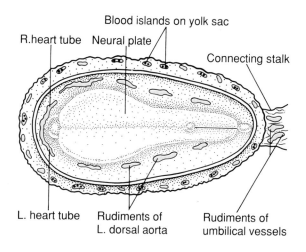

Figure 7.2. Dorsal view of 19-day embryo.

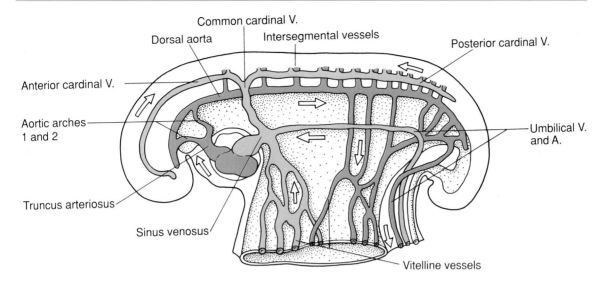

Figure 7.4. Circulatory system at 25 days. Arrows indicate directions of blood flow.

The embryo proper is drained by *interseg- mental veins* which enter paired *anterior* and *posterior cardinal veins* located alongside the dorsal aortas. Paired *common cardinal veins* complete the venous return to the sinus venosus (*Figure 7.4*).

arteries. The arteries enter the chorionic plate and terminate in the capillary bed in the tertiary chorionic villi. Having disposed of waste products and collected oxygen and vital nutrients transferred from the intervil- lous space, the blood returns by way of the umbilical veins to the sinus venosus.

THE EARLY CIRCULATORY SYSTEMS

All of the blood leaving the heart tube reaches the dorsal aortas by way of the trun- cus arteriosus and aortic arch arteries.

Vitelline Circulation

Some of the blood leaves the dorsal aortas by entering the vitelline arteries. Having col- lected red cells from the capillary bed in the wall of the yolk sac, the blood returns in the vitelline veins to the sinus venosus.

Umbilical Circulation

Most of the blood continues caudally in the dorsal aortas before entering the umbilical

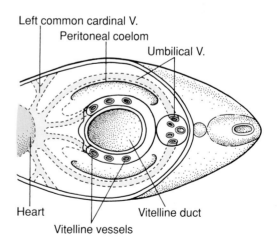

Figure 7.5. Ventral view of 25-day embryo, showing the three sets of embryonic veins.

Embryonic Circulation

An initially small amount of blood enters the tiny intersegmental arteries to nourish the neural tube and the mesodermal somites.

Deoxygenated blood returns to the anterior and posterior cardinal veins, entering the sinus venosus through the two common cardinal veins.

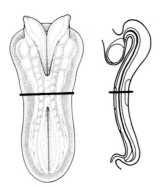

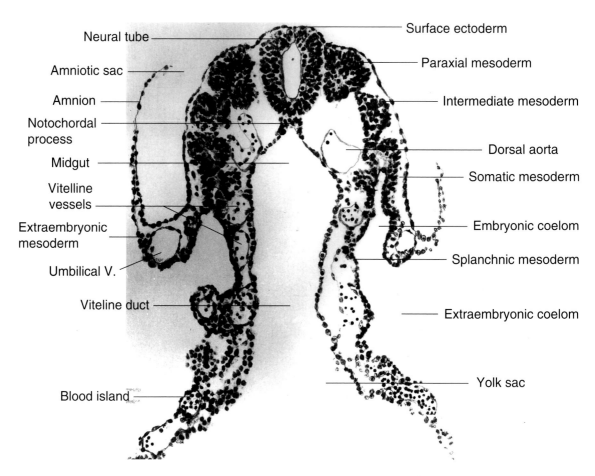

Figure 7.6. Transverse section of a 23-day embryo. (Carnegie Collection.)

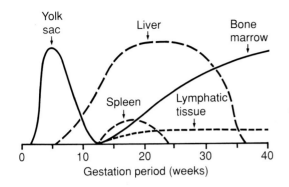

Figure 7.7. Sites and times of hemopoiesis.

HEMOPOIESIS

Formation of embryonic and fetal blood cells passes through three periods, as follows (*Figure 7.7*):

- The *yolk sac period*, extending from week 3 to week 12.

- The *hepatic period*, from week 5 to week 36.

- The *bone marrow period* beginning at the 12th week and continuing throughout the rest of prenatal and postnatal life.

Cells entering the circulation from the blood islands of the yolk sac are nucleated *primitive erythroblasts*. They contain a variant of hemoglobin called hemoglobin F (fetal hemoglobin) which takes up and releases O_2 and CO_2 more readily than adult hemoglobin (hemoglobin A).

In the 5th week, clones of blood-forming cells leave the yolk sac and settle in the spleen. During the 12th week other clones settle in the spleen, bone marrow, thymus and lymph nodes. The red cells produced by the clones in the liver and spleen are more mature than those produced in the wall of the yolk sac, but they still contain a nucleus and hemoglobin F.

Some of the cells settling in the liver, spleen and bone marrow belong to the megakaryocyte and leukocyte series. Those settling in the thymus develop into T lymphocytes. B lymphocytes are formed initially in the liver and spleen and later in lymph nodes.

Non-nucleated erythrocytes of adult type (hemoglobin A) are formed in the bone marrow. During the final month of gestation and throughout postnatal life, erythrocytes are normally formed exclusively in the bone marrow. The short and flat bones and various epiphyses are the main production sites, but in infancy and childhood the marrow in the shafts of the long bones is also red. In adults, although the shaft marrow is white (being fatty), microscopic blood islands remain and they can contribute to erythrocyte production if called upon – for example, in chronic hemorrhagic states.

EMBRYOLOGICAL TERMS

Blood islands. Hemocytoblasts. Angioblasts. Cardiogenic mesoderm. Primitive heart tubes. Primitive heart chambers. Sinus venosus. Truncus arteriosus. Dorsal aorta. Aortic arches. Umbilical arteries and veins. Vitelline arteries and veins. Intersegmental arteries and veins. Anterior, posterior common cardinal veins. Primitive erythroblasts. Hemoglobin F.

8

The embryo at 4 weeks

This chapter presents a description of the anatomy of an embryo 4 weeks old and about 4 mm in length. The objective is to show how the various body systems relate to one another following completion of the folding process.

The embryo is described in the upright position, corresponding to the anatomical position used for description of the postnatal state. Familiar terms of reference have been borrowed from adult anatomy where this has been considered helpful, e.g. above, behind, lower.

SURFACE FEATURES (*Figure 8.1*)

The surface epithelium in the cephalic region shows three thickened areas known as *placodes*.

- The *nasal placode* will become the **olfactory epithelium** lining the roof of the nasal cavity.
- The *lens placode* will form the **lens** of the eye.
- The *otic placode* will form the **membranous labyrinth** of the inner ear.

Four *pharyngeal arches* are seen through the surface in the interval between the brain and the heart. Two more appear during the 5th week. The pharyngeal arches are derived from the paraxial mesoderm. They

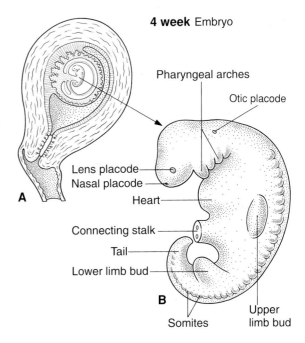

4 week Embryo

Pharyngeal arches
Otic placode
Lens placode
Nasal placode
Heart
Connecting stalk
Tail
Lower limb bud
Somites
Upper limb bud
A
B

Figure 8.1. Four-week embryo. (A) *In utero.* (B) Surface features viewed from left side.

make important contributions to the development of the head and neck.

Some three dozen *somites* can be seen through the surface ectoderm. They are strung like beads along the dorsal aspect of the embryo on each side: 4 occipital, 8 cervical, 12 thoracic, 5 lumbar, 5 sacral, and several coccygeal. (The number of coccygeal somites reaches 8–10 during the 5th week, with full development of the embryonic tail.) The somites are programmed to differentiate into the *myoblasts* that form the skeletal muscles of the trunk; the *osteoblasts* that form the vertebral column; and the *fibroblasts* that form the dermis of the skin.

The *limbs* are blunt projections on the body wall. The upper limb bud is at the level of the lower cervical and uppermost thoracic somites; the lower limb bud is at the level of the lower lumbar and upper sacral somites.

The **heart** is large, because it must sustain three circulatory systems. It is also in a high position at this time in relation to the upper limbs.

DIFFERENTIATION OF THE MESODERM

Figure 8.2 is taken from the dorsal part of the embryo, at the level of the upper limb bud. The following features can be seen in the section and checked against the list in *Table 8.1*:

- The somite has subdivided into three parts: sclerotome, myotome and dermatome. The *sclerotome* is closest to the notochord. As the name implies (Greek, *sclera*, 'hard'), the sclerotomes give rise to bones, namely the **vertebrae**. The

Table 8.1 Derivatives of the embryonic mesoderm

Embryonic mesoderm					
Somites (paraxial mesoderm)			Intermediate mesoderm	Lateral plate mesoderm	
Sclerotomes	Myotomes	Dermatomes		Somatic	Splanchnic
Vertebrae	Muscles of trunk and limbs	Dermis	GUS	Body wall, limb bones and tendons	Heart, mesenteries, smooth muscle of gut

GUS, genitourinary system

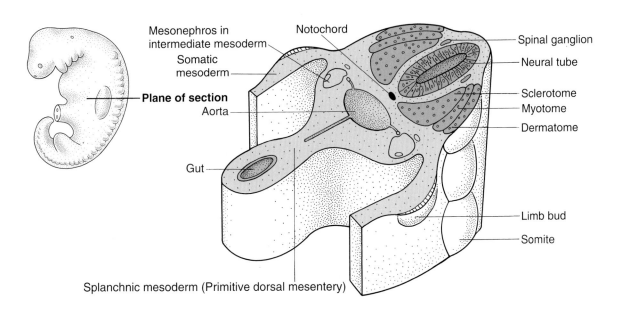

Figure 8.2. Transverse section in the plane indicated at top.

myotomes give rise to the **muscles of the trunk**. The *dermatomes* form the **dermis** of the skin.

- The intermediate mesoderm at this time is forming the *mesonephros* (see Genito-urinary system, later).
- The somatic mesoderm gives rise to the anterior and lateral body wall. The limb buds are outgrowths of the somatic meso-derm. The mesenchyme contained within the buds will form bones and tendons.
  The splanchnic mesoderm of the two sides
- has merged to form a broad *primitive dorsal mesentery* suspending the gut.

Figure 8.3 is a photograph taken from the caudal part of a 4-week embryo.

CIRCULATORY SYSTEM

Arteries

The arterial systems at 25 and 28 days are compared in *Figure 8.4*. The arteries in *Figure 8.4A* are the same as those in *Figure 7.4*.

Four aortic arch arteries are seen in the 4-week embryo. The first and second dis-appear during the 5th week. The third, together with the segment of the dorsal aorta cranial to it, forms the **carotid arterial system**. The fourth artery on the *left* side (shown here) will contribute to the definitive **aortic arch**.

The paired dorsal aortas have fused in the midline (Figure 8.5). Fusion commenced behind the heart and continues down to the

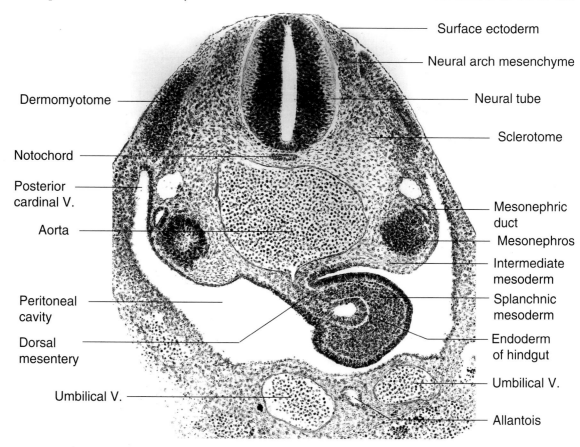

Figure 8.3. Transverse section through the caudal part of a 4-week embryo. (Carnegie Collection.)

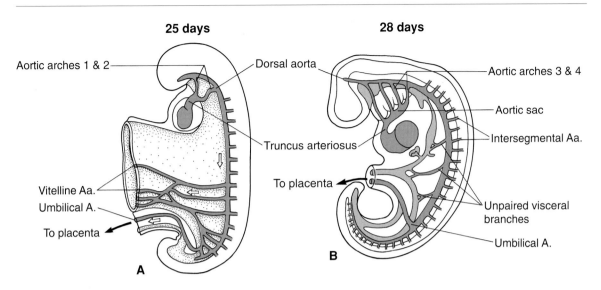

Figure 8.4. Arterial system during the 4th week.

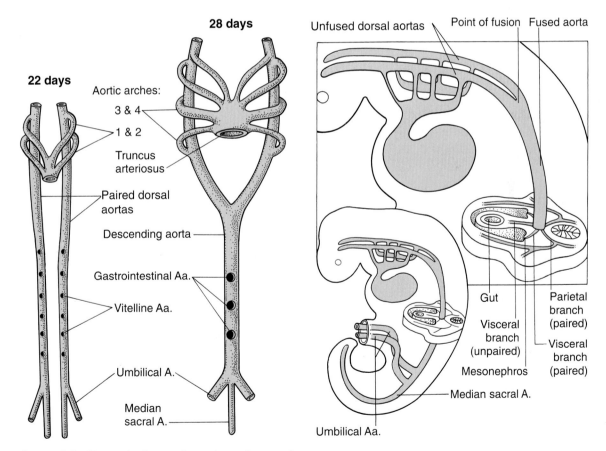

Figure 8.5. Ventral views of aortic arches and dorsal aortas.

Figure 8.6. Details of the dorsal aortas at 4 weeks.

tail end of the embryo. The fused aorta is the forerunner of the **descending thoracic and abdominal aorta** of adult anatomy. During prenatal life the bulk of the circulating blood enters the umbilical arteries, and below this level the aorta persists only as the small **median sacral artery.**

Three sets of branches arise from the fused segment of the aorta (*Figure 8.6*): (a) paired parietal branches supply the neural tube and mesodermal somites; (b) paired visceral branches supply the paired *mesonephroi* (plural of 'mesonephros'); and (c) unpaired visceral branches supply the gut at different levels.

Veins

The venous systems at 25 and 28 days are compared in *Figure 8.7*. The veins are the same as those in *Figure 7.4*.

The *vitelline veins* will be rearranged by the developing liver. They provide the **portal and hepatic veins** of adult anatomy. Of the two *umbilical veins*, only the left persists until birth. The *anterior cardinal veins* become the **internal jugular veins**. The *posterior cardinal veins* contribute to the **inferior caval vein** and to the **azygos** system of veins.

Circulatory Systems

The three circulatory systems of the 4 week embryo are as follows:

- The *vitelline* circulation is represented by the three unpaired visceral arteries and the portal/hepatic veins.
- The *umbilical* circulation is represented by the umbilical arteries, which carry exhausted blood to the placenta, and by the umbilical veins, which return rejuvenated blood to the heart.
- The *embryonic* circulation is represented by intersegmental and cerebral branches of the aorta, and by the corresponding veins draining into the cardinal venous system.

DIGESTIVE SYSTEM

The digestive systems at 25 and 28 days are compared in *Figure 8.8*. At 25 days the

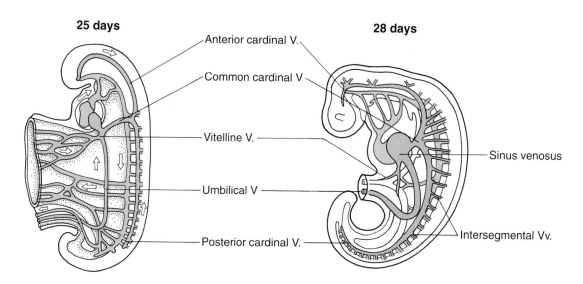

Figure 8.7. Venous system during the 4th week.

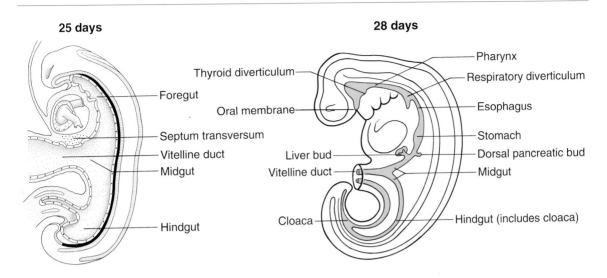

Figure 8.8. Side views of the gut during the 4th week.

foregut reaches from the oral membrane to the rostral limit of the vitelline duct; the midgut faces into the vitelline duct; and the hindgut reaches from the caudal limit of the vitelline duct to the cloacal membrane.

At 28 days the locus of origin of the lower respiratory tract can be identified as the *respiratory (tracheobronchial) diverticulum* of the foregut. The part of the foregut between the oral membrane and the respiratory diverticulum is the *pharynx*. A *thyroid diverticulum* has developed from the pharyngeal endoderm in the midline; it will form the **thyroid gland**.

Caudal to the respiratory diverticulum is a dilatation formed by the **stomach**. The part of the foregut between the respiratory diverticulum and the stomach is the **esophagus**.

Further caudally, a *hepatic diverticulum* (*liver bud*) arises from the endoderm at the point of junction between the fore- and midgut. The liver bud will form the epithelial cells of the **liver** and **gall bladder**. Opposite the liver bud is a *dorsal pancreatic bud*, which will form the bulk of the **pancreas**.

The *midgut* corresponds to the **midgut** of adult anatomy. It will form the **jejunum, ileum** and **proximal colon**.

The *hindgut* will form the **distal colon**. At this time the embryonic hindgut includes the cloaca, which will form the **rectum** and **bladder**.

MESENTERIES AND COELOM

The *primitive dorsal mesentery* encloses the lower end of the esophagus and the gastrointestinal tract. The part behind the lower end of the esophagus is the *mesoesophagus*; the part behind the stomach is the *dorsal mesogastrium*; and the remainder is the *common dorsal mesentery* (*Figure 8.9*).

The *pericardial coelom* encloses the heart, being pierced caudally by the sinus venosus and cranially by the truncus arteriosus. The two sides of the *peritoneal coelom* communicate freely around the vitelline duct, including an extension into the umbilical cord

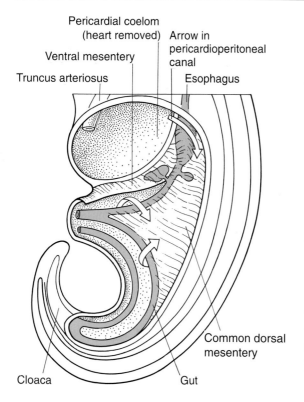

Pericardial coelom
(heart removed)   Arrow in
pericardioperitoneal
canal
Ventral mesentery
Esophagus
Truncus arteriosus

Common dorsal
mesentery

Cloaca   Gut

Figure 8.9. Primitive dorsal mesentery and coelom, viewed from left side. Upper arrow is in pericardioperitoneal canal. Lower arrows indicate continuity of left and right parts of the peritoneal cavity.

(*Figure 8.10*). In the interval between the gut and the dorsal aorta, the two sides are separated by the primitive dorsal mesentery. The *pericardioperitoneal* canals are at the level of the gastroesophageal junction. They are bounded medially by the dorsal mesogastrium and mesoesophagus, laterally by the common cardinal veins, and ventrally by the septum transversum.

GENITOURINARY SYSTEM

The only representatives of the genitourinary system at the end of the 4th week are the *mesonephros* and the *mesonephric duct* (*Figure 8.11*). In females both of these stuctures regress later on. In males, tubules of the mesonephros become the **efferent ductules of the testis** and the mesonephric duct becomes the **ductus (vas) deferens**.

NERVOUS SYSTEM (*Figure 8.12*)

Three *primary brain vesicles* have made their appearance. They are the *forebrain*, *midbrain*,

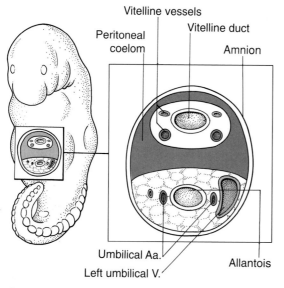

Vitelline vessels
Peritoneal
coelom
Vitelline duct
Amnion

Umbilical Aa.
Left umbilical V.
Allantois

Figure 8.10. The umbilicus at 4 weeks.

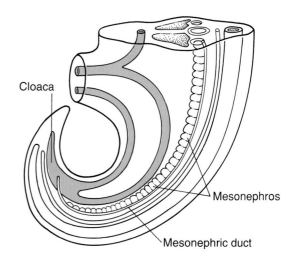

Cloaca

Mesonephros

Mesonephric duct

Figure 8.11. Genitourinary system at 4 weeks.

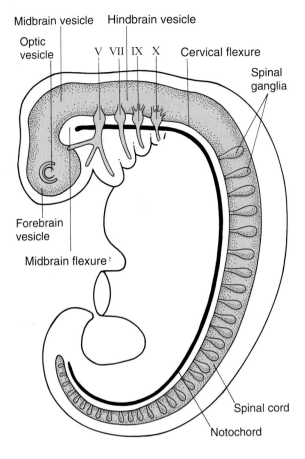

Midbrain vesicle   Hindbrain vesicle

Optic
vesicle   V VII IX X   Cervical flexure

Spinal
ganglia

Forebrain
vesicle

Midbrain flexure

Spinal cord

Notochord

Figure 8.12. Nervous system at 4 weeks. Note sensory ganglia on cranial nerves V (trigeminal), VII (facial), IX (glossopharyngeal) and X (vagus).

and *hindbrain vesicles*. The *optic vesicle* has grown out of the forebrain; it gives rise to the **retina** and **optic nerve**.

Caudal to the brain vesicles, the **spinal cord** is already beginning to differentiate from the epithelium of the neural tube.

The peripheral nerves attached to the brain stem and spinal cord show prominent **sensory ganglia**. They include the **trigeminal ganglion**, the **geniculate ganglion** of the facial nerve, the **sensory ganglia of the glossopharyngeal and vagus**, and the **dorsal root ganglia of the spinal nerves**.

EMBRYOLOGICAL TERMS

Placodes. Pharyngeal arches. Limb buds. Sclerotome. Myotome. Dermatome. Respiratory diverticulum. Hepatic diverticulum (liver bud). Dorsal pancreatic bud. Pharynx. Thyroid diverticulum. Esophagus. Primitive dorsal mesentery. Mesoesophagus. Dorsal mesogastrium. Common dorsal mesentery. Ventral mesogastrium. Mesonephros. Mesonephric duct. Primary brain vesicles. Optic vesicle.

9

Multiple pregnancy

CHAPTER SUMMARY

Twinning
Triplets etc,
Malformations
  Conjoint twins

TWINNING

Twinning occurs in about 1% of pregnancies. Twins are of two kinds: *dizygotic* and *monozygotic*.

Dizygotic twins (sometimes called binovular, or nonidentical) result from fertilization by separate spermatozoa of two simultaneously released ova. The twins may be of the same or of opposite sex, and their genetic endowments are the same as those of ordinary siblings. Binovular twinning shows a hereditary tendency and accounts for 70% of all twins. It is more common in women who have already had one or more children than in first pregnancies.

Each zygote produces its own embryo blast and trophoblast, resulting in two separate individuals each with its own placenta, chorionic sac and amniotic sac.

Monozygotic (monovular) twins develop from a single zygote and have the same genotype. Accordingly, they are of the same sex and resemble each other closely. Their blood groups are the same and their fingerprints are either similar or *enantiomorphic* (mirror images). However, the only absolute proof that they are monovular is the tolerance by one of a tissue graft taken from the other. Monovular twinning is not hereditary and accounts for 30% of all twins.

A single zygote may give rise to twins in three different ways. Examination of fetal membranes (chorion, amnion) after childbirth is usually sufficient to distinguish between them.

Dichorial, diamniotic twins (Figure 9.1A)

In about one-third of identical-twin births, the anatomy of the membranes is the same as that for fraternal twins, with separate chorionic vesicles and amniotic sacs. These babies are the result of separation of blastomeres at the two-cell stage of cleavage. Each of the cells is totipotent, implants separately, and gives rise to a complete individual.

Monochorial, diamniotic twins (Figure 9.1B)

In most identical-twin births, two amniotic sacs develop within a single chorionic vesicle. This form of twinning results from duplication of the embryoblast within a single blastocyst. The trophoblasic shell gives rise to a single placenta in the usual way, and there is a variable degree of anastomosis between the two sets of fetal vessels. Should one take a lion's share, the other will be relatively small at birth. Rarely, one twin is so deprived of access to the maternal vascular bed that it remains very small, is nonviable, and is malformed.

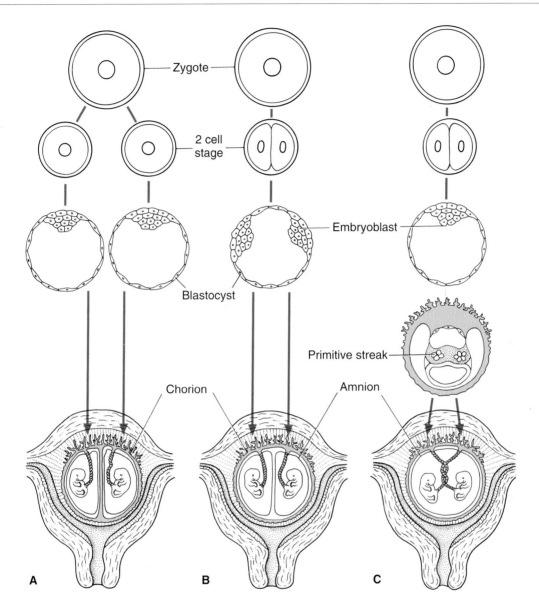

Figure 9.1. Three kinds of twins. (A) Dichorial, diamniotic; (B) monochorial, diamniotic; and (C) monochorial, monoamniotic.

Monochorial, monoamniotic twins (Figure 9.1C)

In about 4% of cases, twinning is delayed until day 14 or 15, at which time a pair of primitive streaks develop side by side. The amniotic sac remains single but the yolk sac is duplicated during formation of the lateral body folds. A major threat to survival is posed by intertwining of the two umbilical cords, with consequent risk of asphyxia.

TRIPLETS ETC.

Triplets may arise in three different ways:

- From a single zygote: separation of blastomeres at the two-cell step (as in *Figure 9.1A*) is followed by a repeat performance by one of the blastomeres, yielding three totipotent cells of identical genetic constitution, three morulas, and three identical babies.
- From two zygotes, one of which yields monozygotic twins.
- From three zygotes, yielding three non-identical siblings of the same or of mixed sexes.

Quintuplets, *sextuplets*, *septuplets*, etc. may arise in the same ways as triplets. Nowadays, much the commonest are nonidentical siblings resulting from multiple ovulation in women of diminished fertility whose ovarian function has been boosted with gonadotropic hormones.

MALFORMATIONS

Conjoint Twins

Conjoint twinning occurs in about 1% of monozygotic twin pregnancies. They all belong to the monochorial, monoamniotic group.

The extent of conjunction is variable: one extreme is represented by a baby containing internal traces of a twin – for example, duplication of the pituitary gland or of the tongue. The other extreme is represented by monozygotic twins joined only by a pedicle of skin. However, two distinct classes are generally recognized:

- Class 1: *Duplex twins*, usually incapable of postnatal survival (*Figure 9.2*). The primitive streak in such cases undergoes *partial* duplication, becoming Y-shaped at one or both ends. The result is a bifurcation of the spinal cord and vertebral column. The

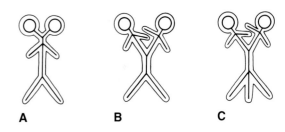

Figure 9.2. Varieties of conjoined twins resulting from incomplete duplication of the primitive streak.

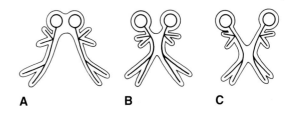

Figure 9.3. Varieties of Siamese twins.

arrangement of the internal organs depends on the extent of the bifurcation of the primitive streak; for example, the conceptus in *Figure 9.2A* would contain one heart whereas that in *Figure 9.2B* would contain two.

- Class 2: *Siamese twins (Figure 9.3)*. Here the duplication is complete with respect to the primitive streak but only partial with respect to the germ layers. Fusion of soft tissues may be rostral, central or caudal, and the twins may be back-to-back, side-to-side, or face-to-face. Surgical separation is usually attempted in centers specializing in such operations.

EMBRYOLOGICAL TERMS

Monozygotic, dizygotic twins. *Conjoint twins. Duplex twins. Siamese twins.*

Regional Embryology

10

Spinal cord

Early in the 4th week, paired neural folds come together as described in Chapter 5, to form the neural tube. The paraxial mesoderm undergoes segmentation to form the somites, and neural crest cells form clusters corresponding to the somites.

Immediately following closure of the caudal neuropore, the neural tube reaches caudally only as far as the second sacral pair of mesodermal somites. The remaining sacral and coccygeal somites differentiate from the paraxial mesoderm during the following week. The corresponding levels of the neural tube develop from the primitive streak by a process known as *secondary neurulation*. An initially solid *neural cord* becomes canalized by caudal extension of the neural canal.

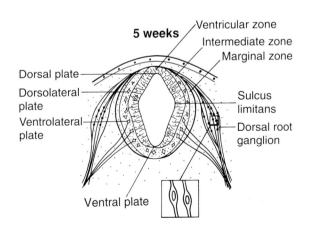

Figure 10.1. Spinal cord at 5 weeks. Dorsal root ganglion cells are bipolar at this time (inset).

PLATES (LAMINAE) OF THE NEURAL TUBE

During the 5th week, a shallow *sulcus limitans* appears on each side of the neural canal (*Figure 10.1*). The side wall dorsal to the sulcus is the *dorsolateral (alar) plate*; the side wall ventral to the sulcus is the *ventrolateral (basal) plate*. In the midline, the *dorsal and ventral (roof and floor) plates* remain thin.

VENTRICULAR, INTERMEDIATE AND MARGINAL ZONES

Three *zones* can be distinguished in the side walls of the neural tube: the ventricular zone, the intermediate zone and the marginal zone.

The *ventricular zone* is next to the neural canal. It is the site of *mitosis* of the neuroepithelial cells (*Figure 10.2*). The nuclei retreat to the base of the cells before they divide. The nuclei of the daughter cells move to the outer part of the ventricular zone where they synthesize DNA before returning to the inner region to divide again.

After several mitotic cycles the daughter cells move out of the ventricular zone. The first cells to move out become neurons (nerve cells) whereas the last to move out become neuroglial cells (connective tissue cells of the central nervous system).

Mitotic activity continues for several weeks, after which time the cells remaining

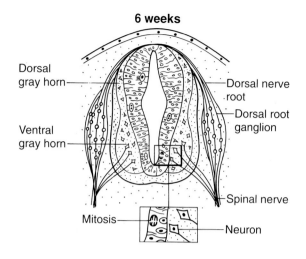

Figure 10.2. Spinal cord at 6 weeks.

in the ventricular zone acquire cilia and become the **ependymal cells** lining the central canal.

The *intermediate (pallial) zone* is the forerunner of the **gray matter** of the spinal cord. It is composed initially of *neuroblasts* that migrate there from the ventricular zone. The neuroblasts differentiate into **neurons** by synthesizing clumps of granular endoplasmic reticulum and emitting processes or **neurites**. Once the process of differentiation begins in neurons, further mitotic activity is impossible.

Glioblasts enter the intermediate zone later. These cells are of two lineages. *Astroblasts* multiply further before differentiating into **astrocytes**; *oligodendroblasts* multiply further before becoming **oligodendrocytes**. Among the functions of astrocytes is provision of structural support for the central nervous system. Oligodendrocytes give rise to myelin sheaths.

A third neuroglial cell type, the phagocytic **microglial cell,** is of mesodermal origin. Microglia originate from the monocytes of the blood. They enter the central nervous system during the third month, by migration from the capillary bed.

The *marginal zone* is the forerunner of the **white matter**. Small neurons are the first to invade the marginal zone. They emit axons alongside the gray matter, establishing **intersegmental pathways** linking different levels of the cord.

During the 6th week (*Figure 10.2*), accumulation of neuroblasts in the dorsolateral plate gives rise to the **dorsal horn** of gray matter, which has a *sensory* function. The dorsal horn receives centrally directed neurites of neural crest cells that accumulate beside the neural tube as **dorsal root ganglia**. The neurons of the dorsal root ganglia are initially *bipolar*, later becoming *unipolar*.

Large accumulations of cells in the ventrolateral plate create the **ventral horn** of gray matter, which has a *motor* function. Axons emerging from the ventral horn form the **ventral nerve roots** of the spinal nerves. The ventral roots join with the peripheral processes of the dorsal root ganglia to form **spinal nerves**.

THE DEFINITIVE SPINAL CORD

During the following 4 weeks (*Figures 10.3 and 10.4*), mitotic activity in the ventricular zone gradually draws to a close, and the *definitive spinal cord* is formed. The neural canal shrinks to become the **central canal** of the spinal cord, and the cells remaining in the ventricular zone become the ciliated **ependymal cells** lining the canal. The **dorsal median septum** develops as a neuroglial partition in the dorsal midline, and the **ventral median fissure** is created by the progressive enlargement of multipolar neurons in the ventral gray horn. A small, **lateral horn** of gray matter develops in the thoracic and upper lumbar segments of the cord (*Figure 10.4*).

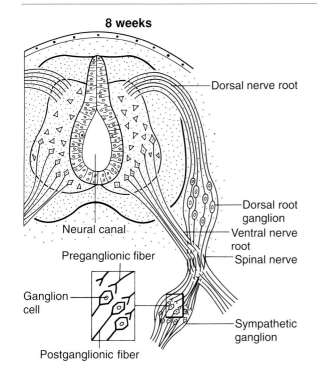

Figure 10.3. Spinal cord and a spinal nerve at 8 weeks.

The centrally directed neurites arising from dorsal root ganglion cells constitute the **dorsal nerve roots** of the respective spinal nerves. The larger neurites give collateral branches that ascend in the dorsal part of the marginal zone. These will form the fast-conducting **dorsal funiculi (posterior columns)** of white matter when they acquire myelin sheaths. The peripherally directed neurites of dorsal root ganglion cells terminate in sensory nerve endings in the body wall, limbs and viscera. The **lateral** and **ventral funiculi** of white matter are formed by ascending pathways originating in the neurons of the dorsal gray horn, and by descending pathways originating at various levels of the brain.

THE CELL COLUMNS OF THE SPINAL CORD

Four cell columns are described as follows (*Figure 10.4*):

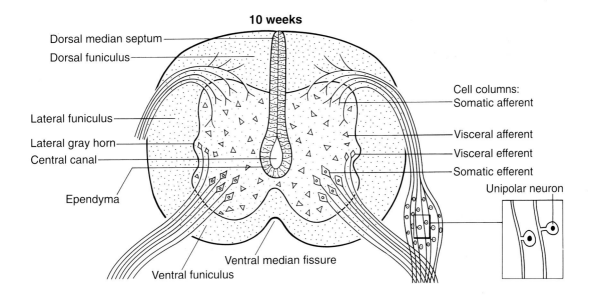

Figure 10.4. Spinal cord at 10 weeks. Inset: Dorsal root ganglion cells are becoming unipolar.

In the ventrolateral plate,

- a *somatic efferent cell column* supplies skeletal muscle in the trunk and limbs;
- a *visceral efferent cell column* sends sympathetic preganglionic fibers into the ventral nerve roots at thoracic and upper lumbar segmental levels, and parasympathetic preganglionic fibers into the ventral roots at mid-sacral level.

In the dorsolateral plate,

- a *visceral afferent cell column* belongs to the afferent limb of visceral reflex arcs;
- a *somatic afferent cell column* receives afferent fibers from skin, skeletal muscles and joints.

Ascent of the spinal cord within the vertebral canal is described in Chapter 11, along with the filum terminale and cauda equina.

FATE OF THE NEURAL CREST

The neural crest is *pluripotent*, being able to form tissues of more than one type. In the head region, in particular, many neural crest cells become *mesectoderm*, contributing cells to tissues that originate from the mesoderm in other regions.

The following cell types and tissues are generally agreed to originate from the neural crest:

1. The dorsal root ganglion cells of the spinal nerves.
2. Autonomic ganglion cells.
3. The chromaffin cells of the adrenal medulla. The chromaffin cells are modified sympathetic neuroblasts.
4. The sheath cells of peripheral nerves, namely the satellite cells of dorsal root ganglia, Schwann cells distributed along the nerves, and the teloglial cells investing some sensory nerve endings (notably the highly sensitive Meissner's and Pacinian corpuscles). The Schwann cells form the myelin sheaths investing all but the finest axons of the peripheral nerves. (Histology or neuroanatomy texts should be consulted for details of the myelination process.)
5. The pia-arachnoid sheath enclosing the subarachnoid space around the brain and spinal cord.
6. The melanocytes of the skin. Precursor cells originate from the neural crest and migrate along the peripheral nerves to reach the skin.
7. The connective tissue in the wall of the outflow tract of the embryonic heart and of the great arteries (Chapter 13).
8. Parafollicular cells of the thyroid gland, and the glomus cells of the carotid and aortic bodies (Chapter 25).
9. Much of the craniofacial skeleton (Chapter 26)
10. The *odontoblasts* of the developing teeth (Chapter 26).

MALFORMATIONS

Because the vertebral column is involved as well, congenital malformations of the spinal cord are described in the next chapter.

EMBRYOLOGICAL TERMS

Neuroepithelial cells. Secondary neurulation. Neural cord. Sulcus limitans. Dorsolateral and ventrolateral plates, dorsal and ventral plates. Ventricular, intermediate and marginal zones. Glioblasts. Astroblasts. Oligodendroblasts. Mesectoderm. Melanoblasts. Odontoblasts.

11
Body wall including vertebral column

SKELETAL STRUCTURES: VERTEBRAL COLUMN

Four phases can be identified in the development of the vertebral column: mesenchymal, blastemal, cartilaginous and bony.

Mesenchymal Vertebral Column

The precursors of the vertebrae are the paired *sclerotomes*, which are derived from the medial parts of the somites. The sclerotomes consist of branched mesenchymal cells. They surround the notochord and form a *mesenchymal vertebral column* (*Figure 11.1A*). The mesenchymal vertebrae are segmented because the parent somites constitute the body segments. The spinal nerves enter the dermomyotomes whereas the intersegmental vessels pass between the vertebrae.

Blastemal Phase

The rostral half of each mesenchymal vertebra has a 'rarified' appearance because of the relative sparsity of cells. The caudal half is relatively 'condensed.' The cells at the interface between the rostral and caudal halves form an **intervertebral disc**. The remainder of the condensed element *merges with the vertebra caudal to it* (*Figure 11.1B*). In this manner the *centrum* (main part) of a *blastemal* vertebra is formed from two sclerotomes on each side.

From the condensed upper part of the centrum, a pair of *neural arches* grows dorsally to embrace the neural tube. A notch near the commencement of the neural arch accommodates intersegmental vessels supplying the spinal cord (*Figure 11.2A*). The notch deepens to take in the spinal nerve as well. In this way the spinal vessels and nerve come to occupy the **intervertebral foramen**, located between the **pedicles** of the vertebrae above and below. These relationships are shown for the mature vertebral column in *Figure 11.2B*.

The blastemal neural arches give rise to paired *costal* and *transverse processes* (*Figure 11.3A*). Finally, the arches unite in the dorsal midline where they produce *spinous processes* (*Figure 11.3B*).

Cartilaginous Phase

The blastemal vertebral column becomes cartilaginous, following the appearance of chondrification centers in the centrum and neural arch late in the 5th week (*Figure 11.3A*). In the case of the 12 thoracic vertebrae, the cartilaginous costal processes

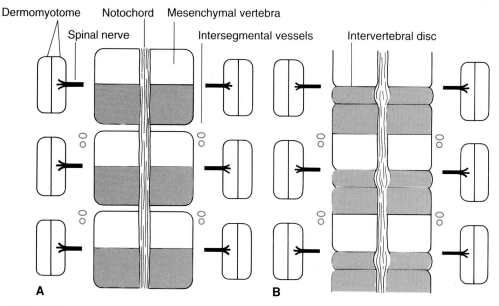

Figure 11.1. Schematic coronal sections of (A) mesenchymal vertebrae, (B) blastemal vertebrae.

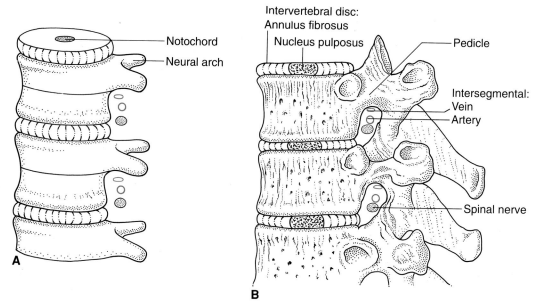

Figure 11.2. (A) Side view of blastemal vertebrae. (B) Schematic section of adult vertebrae showing contents of two intervertebral for amina.

become detached from the parent neural arches by the establishment of synovial joints (*Figure 11.3B*). Synovial joints are also created between the costal and transverse processes (*Figure 11.4*).

At other levels, the costal processes are incorporated into the vertebrae. The costal elements of mature cervical, lumbar and sacral vertebrae are shown in *Figure 11.5*.

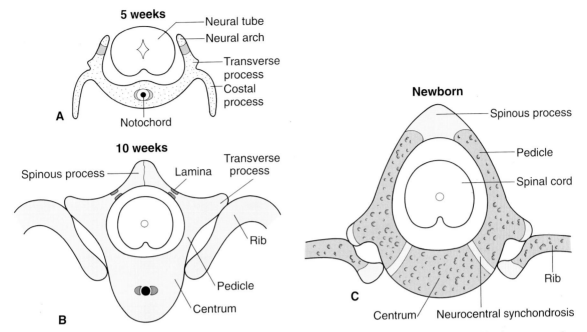

Figure 11.3 (A). Blastemal vertebra with centers of chondrification (in blue). (B) Cartilaginous vertebra with centers of ossification (in red). (C) Bony vertebra.

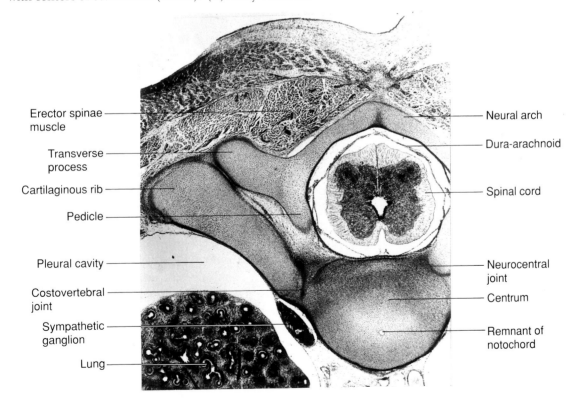

Figure 11.4. Posterior wall of thorax at 10 weeks. (Carnegie Collection.)

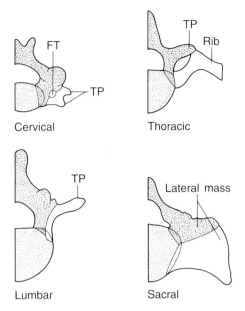

Cervical   Thoracic

Lumbar   Sacral

Figure 11.5. Centrum (light stipple), neural arch (heavy stipple), and costal element (black) at different vertebral levels. FT, foramen transversarium; TP, the transverse process of descriptive anatomy.

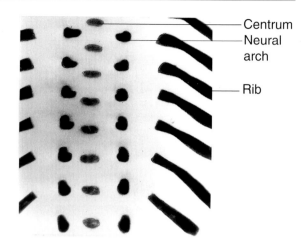

Figure 11.6. Alizarin-stained thoracic vertebrae and ribs, showing extent of ossification at 12 weeks.

Bony Phase

In the 8th week, ossification centers appear in the cartilaginous centra and neural arches, and in the ribs (*Figure 11.3B*). These centers are well defined at 12 weeks (*Figure 11.6*). The vertebrae and ribs are extensively ossified before birth. Until the second postnatal year, cartilaginous plates known as *neurocentral synchondroses* are located at the junctions of the neural arches with the centra (*Figure 11.3C*). The **bodies** of the definitive vertebrae include the centra together with the roots of the neural arches.

The notochord disappears from the centra, but within the intervertebral discs it enlarges to form the gelatinous **nucleus pulposus**. The cellular condensation that defined the position of the discs undergoes fibrocartilaginous change to form the surrounding **annulus fibrosus** of the disc.

Meninges

The meninges are laid down during the blastemal period. Cells shed from the inside rim of the neural arches form the fibrous **dura mater** lining the vertebral canal. The delicate **pia-arachnoid** is formed by neural crest cells.

Ascent of the Spinal Cord

The spinal cord initially occupies the full length of the vertebral canal including the *embryonic tail* derived from 8–10 coccygeal sclerotomes (*Figure 11.7A*). During the 7th and 8th weeks, the tail undergoes *regression*, with reduction of the embryonic coccygeal vertebrae to only three. The enclosed part of the neural tube shrinks as well, dwindling to a neuroglial thread, the **filum terminale** (*Figure 11.7B*).

After the 12th week the vertebral column grows more rapidly than the spinal cord, and the cord is forced to ascend the vertebral canal (*Figure 11.7C*). The tip of the cord

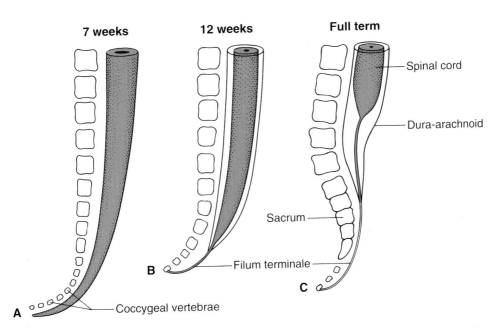

Figure 11.7. (A, B) Formation of filum terminale. (C) Ascent of spinal cord. Sacral vertebrae are shaded.

reaches the second or third lumbar level at the time of birth. The adult level (first or second lumbar) is reached 3 weeks later.

Varying degrees of obliquity are imposed upon the spinal nerve roots because they are anchored proximally to the cord and distally to the intervertebral foramina (*Figure 11.8*). The first cervical roots are an exception, because spinal nerve C1 emerges between the atlas and the skull. Ascent of all of the remaining segments has an additive effect from above downward, with the effect of producing an increasing disparity between spinal segmental levels and vertebral levels. (A spinal segment is defined as the segment of the cord to which a given pair of nerve roots is attached.)

The nerve roots descending below the tapered tip of the cord form the **cauda equina** (Latin, 'horse's tail'). The full complement of nerve roots in the upper end of the cauda equina is 40: lowest 4 lumbar, 5 sacral, 1 coccygeal, all ×4 to account for the dorsal and ventral roots of right and left sides.

SKELETAL STRUCTURES: RIBS AND STERNUM

During the 4th week the **umbilicus** is created by the ventral progression of the lateral body folds (*Figure 11.9A,B*). The somatic mesoderm of the lateral folds is penetrated by the thoracic costal processes, which induce the somatic mesoderm to add to their tips, and in this way to complete the formation of the blastemal ribs.

The **sternum** originates in the form of two *sternal bars* in the ventral part of the somatic mesoderm (*Figure 11.9C*). The two bars meet in the midline in the shape of an inverted V, and they unite from above downward to form a mesenchymatous **sternum**. Except in rare cases of *cleft sternum*, the two halves of the **manubrium** and **body** unite successfully,

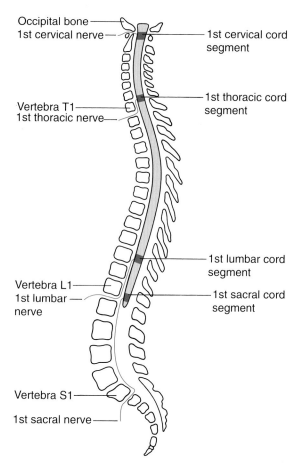

Figure 11.8. Effects of spinal cord ascent upon the course of nerve roots within the mature vertebral canal.

but the **xiphisternum** often remains permanently bifid. The ventral ends of the rostral seven costal processes fuse with the sternum, all but the first being later separated from it by tiny synovial joints.

The sternum and ribs undergo cartilaginous transformation and subsequent ossification, with the exception of the ventral ends of the costal processes which persist as the **costal cartilages**.

SOFT TISSUES

The *dermomyotomes* are what remain of the somites after the sclerotomes depart to surround the notochord. During formation of the lateral body folds, the dermomyotomes split into the component *myotomes* and *dermatomes*.

Myotomes

The myotomes give rise to the **muscles of the neck and trunk**. Included here are the muscles linking the vertebrae to one another and to the skull, together with the muscles of the thoracic and abdominal walls. *Excluded* are the sternomastoid and trapezius, along with muscles that develop within the upper limb and gain secondary attachment to the trunk (latissimus dorsi, pectoralis major and minor, rhomboids, serratus anterior).

Each myotome first divides into a dorsal *epimere* and a ventral *hypomere* (*Figure 11.10*). The corresponding spinal nerve divides into **dorsal and ventral rami** to supply the muscles with motor fibers originating in the ventral horn of the cord. The overlying dermatome (as well as the muscles) is supplied (via the rami) with sensory fibers originating in a dorsal root ganglion.

The epimeres lose most of their segmental character by linking longitudinally to form the **erector spinae** muscle mass.

The hypomeres migrate into the lateral plate mesoderm along with the dermatomes and the ventral rami of the spinal nerves. Body wall muscles differentiate from the hypomeres in three primary layers, the ventral rami occupying the interval between the middle and the inner layer (*Figure 11.10*). The external layer forms the **scalenus posterior** in the neck, the **external intercostals** in the thorax, and the **external oblique** in

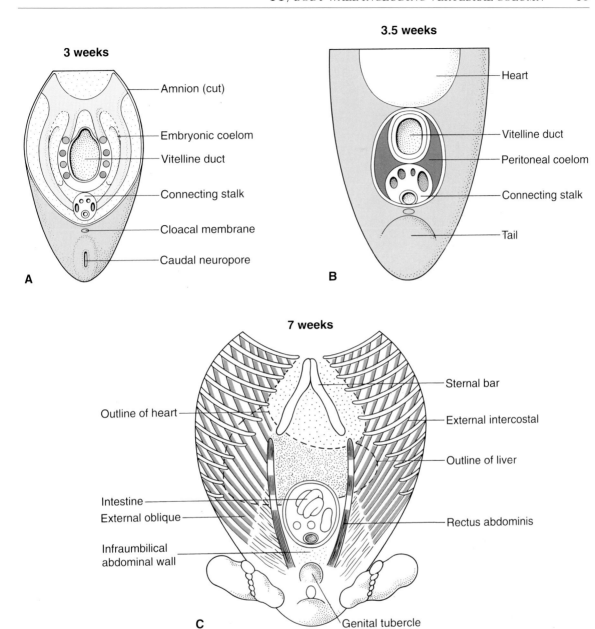

Figure 11.9. Embryonic abdominal wall.

the abdomen (*Figure 11.9*). The middle layer forms the **scalenus medius, internal intercostals** and **internal oblique**. The innermost layer forms the **scalenus anterior, subcostals** and **transversus abdominis**. It also forms the **quadratus lumborum** and **levator ani**.

The **rectus abdominis** represents the most ventral extension of the myotomes. Its multisegmental origin is indicated by its

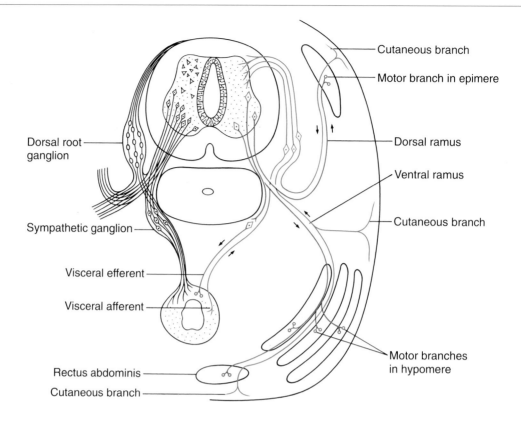

Dorsal root ganglion

Sympathetic ganglion

Visceral efferent

Visceral afferent

Rectus abdominis

Cutaneous branch

Cutaneous branch

Motor branch in epimere

Dorsal ramus

Ventral ramus

Cutaneous branch

Motor branches in hypomere

Figure 11.10. Component elements of an embryonic thoracic spinal nerve. The bipolar dorsal root ganglion cells become unipolar during the 10th week.

nerve supply from the lower six thoracic and first lumbar nerves, and by the occurrence of **tendinous intersections** traversing the muscle above (and sometimes below) the umbilicus.

Dermatomes

The dermatomes merge with one another and permeate the somatic mesoderm of the lateral and anterior body wall (*Figure 11.11*). They form the connective tissue layer or **dermis** of the skin. Each dermatome is accompanied during its migration by sensory nerve fibers derived from the spinal nerve at that level. In this way the dermatomes of clinical neurology are formed.

The clinical 'dermatome' is the band of skin supplied by an individual spinal nerve. The clinical dermatomes overlap with one another in the sense that a given spinal nerve supplies part of the dermatomes immediately rostral and caudal as well as its own one.

The **infraumbilical abdominal wall** seems to be distinctive in acquiring a contribution from the caudal mesoderm. Formation of the tail fold carries the caudal mesoderm to the ventral aspect of the embryo. Here it contributes to the external genitalia in the form of a *genital tubercle* (*Figure 11.9*). It spreads rostrally into the somatic mesoderm, displacing the allantois and umbilical vessels ahead of it.

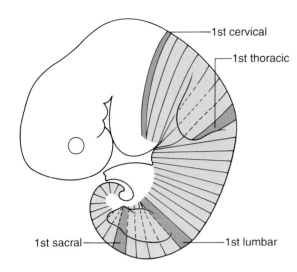

Figure 11.11. Dermatomes, early in the 5th week.

Fate of the Intersegmental Arteries

Cervical intersegmental arteries disappear because their territory is taken over by the vertebral artery. *Thoracic* intersegmental arteries become **intercostal arteries**. *Lumbar* intersegmental arteries become **lumbar arteries**. Sacral intersegmental arteries become the **lateral sacral** branches of the internal iliac artery.

The Skin and the Mammary Gland

Skin

The epidermis and the skin appendages are derived from the surface ectoderm. The connective tissue of the dermis develops from the dermatomes, following migration of the dermatomes through the scaffolding provided by the somatic mesoderm.

The surface ectoderm is initially cuboidal. During the second month it becomes two-layered. The superficial layer (known as *periderm*) is shed. The remaining, *germinal* layer forms the epithelial structures of the skin.

During the third month, (a) the germinal layer gives rise to the stratified squamous epithelium of the **epidermis**; (b) the basal layer of the epidermis sends epithelial pegs into the dermis, forming the epithelial root sheath of **hair follicles**; and (c) the dermis responds by contributing the dermal root sheath and the capillary loops within the hair bulb. During the fifth month the **sebaceous glands** bud into the dermis from the outer root sheath, and the **sweat glands** grow down from the epidermis.

The first, fine coat of hair formed over the body surface is called *lanugo*. The *vernix caseosa* ('cheesy varnish') is a sebaceous secretion, mixed with peridermal cells and lanugo hairs, covering the body during fetal life and obvious on the newborn baby as a whitish paste. The vernix protects the skin from the macerating effect of amniotic fluid and provides some thermal insulation immediately after birth.

The lanugo hair is shed shortly before or after birth, to be succeeded by coarser, *vellus* hair. The vellus hair is largely derived from a second set of hair follicles that replaces the first.

Mammary Gland

In the 6th week, a strip of ectodermal thickening, the *mammary ridge*, extends from the axilla to the groin on each side. Normally, a single **breast** develops from the thoracic part of the ridge, and the remainder of the ridge disappears. The breast develops by an inward sprouting of about 20 epithelial cords that become canalized to form **lactiferous ducts**. The original ectodermal thickening becomes depressed until the perinatal period, when it rises to form the **nipple**. In girls, glandular acini develop from the duct system at puberty. However, some acini may be already present before birth, and lactogenic hormone may cross the placenta from the maternal blood and cause secretion of so-called 'witch's milk' for a few days after birth.

MALFORMATIONS

Spina bifida

The term 'spina bifida' owes its origin to a failure of the neural arches to unite behind the spinal cord. The bifid (split) elements are the separated pairs of vertebral laminae (*Figure 11.12A*). The condition usually occurs in the lumbosacral region. In its simplest form, the defect is seen on routine radiological examination. This is *spina bifida occulta*, a minor anomaly occurring in 1% of the population.

Spina bifida cystica belongs to an important group of malformations classified under the general heading, *neural tube defects* (NTDs). NTDs include some major malformations of the brain, notably *anencephaly* (absence of the cerebral hemispheres) and *hydrocephalus* (ballooning of the cerebral ventricles caused by obstruction of cerebrospinal fluid circulation). Brain malformations are described in Chapter 30.

Three variants of spina bifida cystica are described. About 10% of cases are *meningoceles* (*Figure 11.12B*). Here the meninges protrude as a cyst beneath the intact skin, and the nervous system is usually unimpaired. The remaining 90% are either *meningomyeloceles* or *myeloceles*. In the former (*Figure 11.12C*), the spinal cord or cauda equina floats within a meningeal cyst, and the overlying skin is extremely thin (*Figure 11.13*). Neurological deficits in the lower limbs are the rule, together with incontinence of the bladder and rectum. In addition, most infants with meningomyelocele have some degree of hydrocephalus. With myeloceles (also called *rachischisis*), the neural tube has failed to close in the lumbar region (*Figure 11.12D*), and cerebrospinal fluid oozes over an open trough of neural tissue. The lower limbs and pelvic organs are paralyzed, and

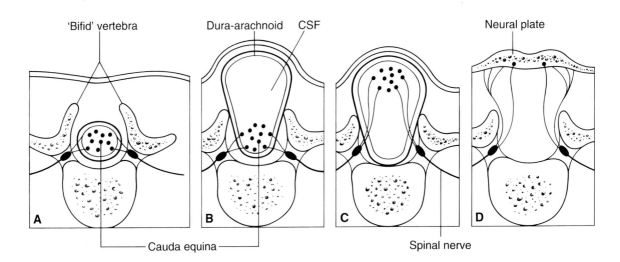

Figure 11.12. Variants of spina bifida. (A) Spina bifida occulta. (B) Meningocele. (C), Meningomyelocele. (D) Myelocele.

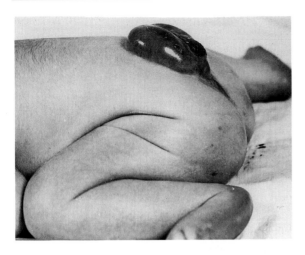

Figure 11.13. Meningomyelocele. The 'frog leg' posture is characteristic of combined femoral and sciatic nerve paralysis, with preservation of hip flexion by the iliopsoas muscles. (Photograph kindly supplied by Dr F. W. F. Kerr, Mayo Clinic, Rochester, Minnesota, USA.)

death ultimately follows infection of the nervous or urinary system.

NTDs, with their frequent concurrence of cerebral and spinal defects, account for about 10% of all congenital malformations. Epidemiological studies indicate a mild genetic predisposition, and a significant relationship to malnutrition. A normal or above-normal dietary intake of folic acid affords significant protection in susceptible populations. For example, in Dublin, Ireland the annual incidence fell from 6.2 per 1000 births in 1975, to 2.3 per 1000 in 1987 – a dramatic decline, attributed in the main to consumption of breakfast cereals fortified with folic acid.

Other Skeletal Anomalies

Variations in the number of vertebrae are not uncommon. Most frequent are *sacralization* of the fifth lumbar vertebra (giving rise to a sacrum with six vertebrae instead of the usual five); and *lumbarization* of the first sacral vertebra.

A pair of *supernumerary ribs* may result from elongation of lower cervical or upper lumbar costal processes during development. A *cervical rib* is especially significant because it may produce severe effects during adult life. It takes the form of a strand of bone or of fibrous tissue, extending from the seventh cervical transverse process to the medial border of the first rib. It may elevate the lower trunk of the brachial plexus, causing motor, sensory and/or autonomic symptoms in the hand (e.g. paralysis of intrinsic muscles, ulnar pain, swelling and redness).

Mammary Glands

Polythelia (one or more supernumerary nipples) may occur anywhere along the mammary ridge from axilla to groin. Rudimentary breasts may develop from them (*polymastia*). Very rarely, nipples (and therefore breasts) fail to appear at all (*athelia*).

EMBRYOLOGICAL TERMS

Sclerotome. Blastemal vertebra. Centrum. Neural arch. Dermomyotome. Myotome. Dermatome. Costal process. Embryonic tail. Sternal bars. Genital tubercle. Epimere. Hypomere. Periderm. Lanugo. Vernix caseosa. Vellus hair. Mammary ridge. *Spina bifida occulta. Spina bifida cystica. Neural tube defects (NTDs). Anencephaly. Hydrocephaly. Meningocele. Meningomyelocele. Myelocele (rachischisis). Sacralization of LV5. Lumbarization of SV1. Polythelia. Polymastia. Athelia.*

12

The limbs

The limbs are formed from the somatic mesoderm of the lateral body wall. Minute *upper limb buds* appear in the middle of the 4th week, at the level of the lower cervical somites (*Figure 12.1*). The *lower limb buds* appear about 2 days later, at the level of the lower lumbar somites. Throughout the prenatal period, the main phases of upper limb development are a few days in advance of those of the lower limbs.

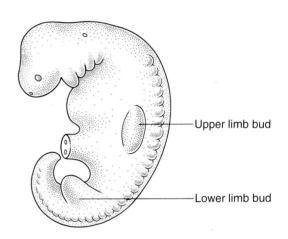

Figure 12.1. Limb buds at 4 weeks.

APICAL ECTODERMAL RIDGE. PROGRESS ZONE

At the level of each limb bud, proliferation of somatic mesodermal cells is induced by an *apical ectodermal ridge* (AER). The AER is formed by thickening of the surface ectoderm, initially over the bud as a whole (*Figure 12.2*) but later only at the growing tip (*Figure 12.3*). The bud is filled with loose mesenchyme. Mitotic activity in the mesenchyme is virtually restricted to a *progress zone* immediately deep to the AER. Daughter cells separate out from the progress zone and they increase the length of the limb by adding to the cell population at the apex of the bud. The mesenchyme is permeated by capillaries which drain into a prominent *marginal vein* close to the progress zone.

In experimental animals, removal of the AER from an early forelimb bud is followed by cessation of all mitotic activity in progress zone. The mesoderm in such cases differentiates into proximal structures including the bones and muscles of the limb girdle (scapula, clavicle) while the distal part of the limb does not develop.

FORMATION OF HANDS AND FEET

During the 5th week, the primordia of the hands and feet become apparent in the form of flat *limb plates* (*Figure 12.4*). The AER is at first arranged in a strip along the distal edge of each plate, before breaking up into five ridges marking the future position of the digits (*Figure 12.5*). The five cell clusters are, in fact, responsible for formation of the digits, because each one induces and maintains a progress zone which in turn lays down a

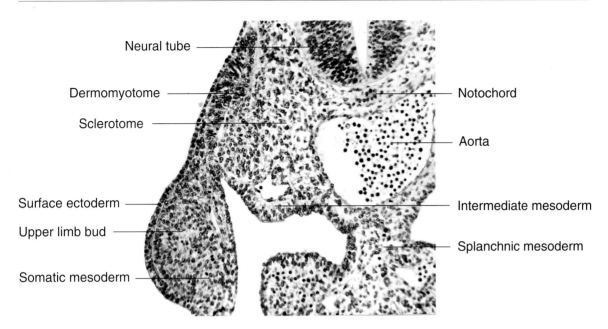

Figure 12.2. Transverse section of a 4-week embryo, at the level of the upper limb bud. (Cambridge Collection.)

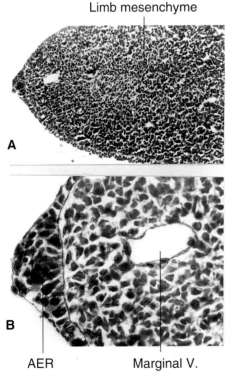

Figure 12.3. (A) Upper limb bud at 5 weeks. (B) Enlargement from (A); AER, apical ectodermal ridge.

rod of mesoderm. The five rods are sometimes called *digital rays*.

The intervals between the digital rays are occupied at first by webs of loose mesenchyme. While the digits are developing, the webs undergo *programmed cell death* to create the *interdigital clefts*.

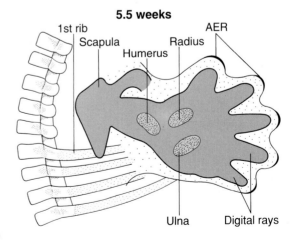

Figure 12.4. Transilluminated 6-week embryo.

ROTATION OF THE LIMBS

During the 8th week, the limbs undergo *rotation*, in a manner that could be predicted from the adult arrangement of the limb segments. At the beginning of that week, the pollux (thumb) and hallux (big toe) regions have a rostral position within the limb plates, and the knee and elbow regions face outward (*Figure 12.6A*). As the week progresses, elbow and knee creases appear. The upper limb then rotates dorsally, carrying the point of the elbow to the back and the pollux to the lateral side. The lower limb rotates ventrally, carrying the point of the knee to the front and the hallux to the medial side (*Figure 12.6B*).

LIMB SKELETON

Just like the vertebral column, the skeleton of the limbs passes through blastemal and cartilaginous stages before undergoing endochondral ossification. A notable single exception is the **clavicle**, in which the blastemal model undergoes intramembranous ossification.

During the 5th week, condensations of the limb mesenchyme form a *blastemal skeleton* which gives only a rough outline of the limb

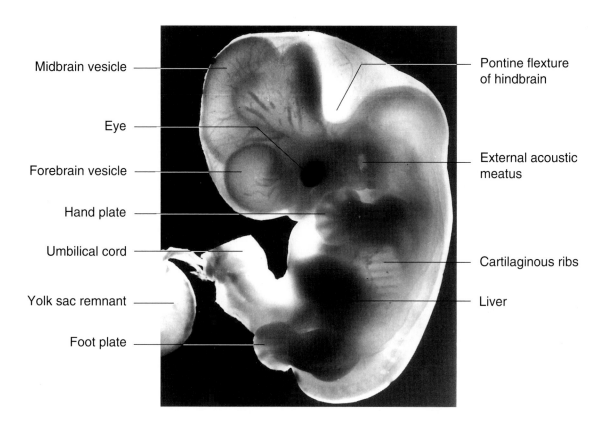

Figure 12.5. Blastemal model of the upper limb skeleton at 5½ weeks, with centers of chondrification shown in blue. AER, apical ectodermal ridge.

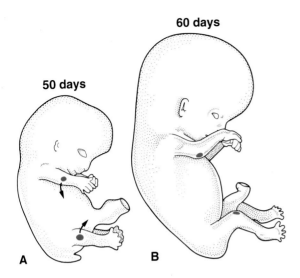

Figure 12.6. Positions of the extensor aspects (red marks) of elbow and knee, (A) before and (B) after rotation of the limbs.

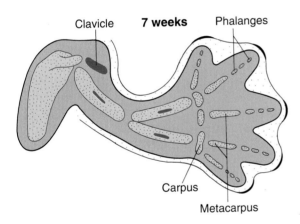

Figure 12.7. Upper limb skeleton at 7 weeks. Centers of ossification (red) have appeared in the clavicle and in the three major long bones.

skeleton (*Figure 12.5*). By the end of the 7th week, the blastemal tissue has been converted into cartilage, and centers of ossification have appeared in the three major long bones (*Figure 12.7*). By the end of the 12th week (*Figure 12.8*), ossification is well advanced in the major long bones and has begun in the minor long bones (metacarpals and metatarsals, phalanges). In the tarsus,

ossification of the three largest bones (calcaneus, talus, cuboid) commences in late fetal life, but the carpus remains cartilaginous until after birth.

MUSCLES AND NERVES

Evidence from experimental embryology indicates that the striated musculature of the limbs differentiates from cells that migrate into the limb buds from the nearest somites. Tendons, on the other hand, seem to differentiate from somatic mesoderm already contained within the buds.

At first, the upper and lower limb buds are relatively rostrally placed; for example, the scapular condensation is above the level of the first rib (*Figure 12.4*). Before they descend to their final position, the limbs are invaded by the ventral rami of the adjacent spinal nerves – the upper limb by nerves C5–T1, the lower limb by nerves L2–S2.

The ventral rami are mixed nerves. They carry motor fibers from the ventral gray horn of the spinal cord, and sensory fibers from dorsal root ganglia. They make contact with groups of myoblasts near the limb roots, and here the ventral rami branch and interconnect to form the brachial and lumbosacral plexuses. The nerve trunks issuing from the plexuses are also mixed, providing motor and sensory fibers to the musculature and sensory fibers to the skin. There appears to be some distal migration of the skin relative to the musculature because the cutaneous territories of the nerve trunks finally lie distal to the motor territories (the musculocutaneous, radial, femoral, and tibial nerves are clear examples). The cutaneous branches seen in gross dissections are derived from dorsal root ganglia that contribute to two or more segments of the spinal cord. The dermis develops *in situ* from the

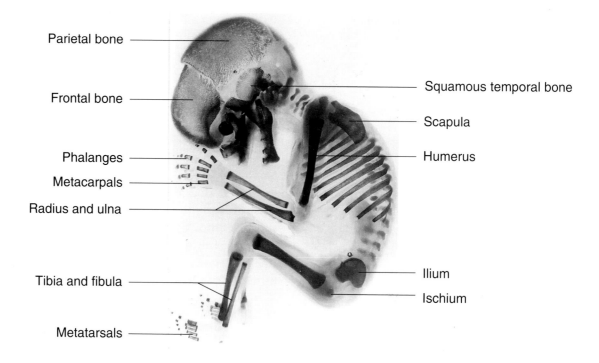

Labels on figure: Parietal bone, Frontal bone, Phalanges, Metacarpals, Radius and ulna, Tibia and fibula, Metatarsals, Squamous temporal bone, Scapula, Humerus, Ilium, Ischium

Figure 12.8. Alizarin-stained skeleton at 16 weeks.

somatic mesoderm, and the neurological dermatomes are surprisingly well-ordered in spite of the interconnections occurring in the limb plexuses (*Figure 12.9*).

BLOOD SUPPLY

The early limb buds are invaded by branches of the intersegmental vessels, and these provide a rich capillary network throughout the limb mesenchyme. The arterial supply resolves into a single *axial artery* running through the core of the limb (*Figure 12.10A*). The distal capillary bed drains into a *marginal vein* close to the AER. More proximal capillaries drain into a *preaxial vein* running along the rostral border of the limb, and into a *postaxial vein* along the caudal border. Following rotation of the limbs. the preaxial veins can be identified as the **cephalic vein** in the upper limb and the **great saphenous vein** in the lower limb; the corresponding postaxial veins are the basilic vein and the **short saphenous vein**.

The developing limb skeleton displaces the axial arteries, and these are replaced to a significant extent by new vessels (*Figure 12.10B,C*). In the upper limb, the **axillary, brachial and anterior interosseous arteries** represent the original axial artery. The **radial and ulnar arteries** sprout from the brachial and take over the supply to the forearm and hand. In the lower limb, the **inferior gluteal artery** and its sciatic branch, and the **popliteal and peroneal arteries** are remnants of the axial artery. The **femoral artery** invades the lower limb as a new vessel that joins the popliteal artery. The **anterior and posterior tibial arteries** – new vessels homologous with the radial and ulnar – sprout from the popliteal and supply the leg and foot.

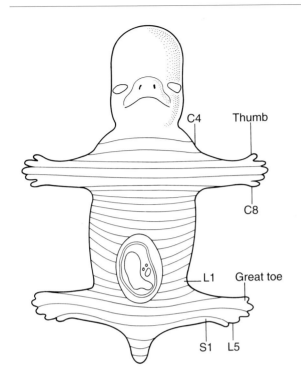

Figure 12.9. Embryonic dermatome pattern.

MALFORMATIONS

Serious malformations of the limbs are rare, and usually hereditary. Drugs are seldom the cause, because the thalidomide disaster in the early 1960s highlighted the risk of taking *any* kind of drug during the 6th to 10th week of pregnancy (4th to 8th week of development). (Thalidomide, used to control morning sickness in early pregnancy, caused thousands of cases of major limb malformations. Humans were much more susceptible than the laboratory animals used for initial screening of the drug.)

Complete failure of the limbs to develop is *amelia* (*Figure 12.11A*). Failure of proximal limb segments with more or less successful development of distal parts is *meromelia* (*Figure 12.11B*). *Syndactyly* is a fusion of two fingers or toes (*Figure 12.11C*); usually, only soft tissues are involved. *Polydactyly* is the

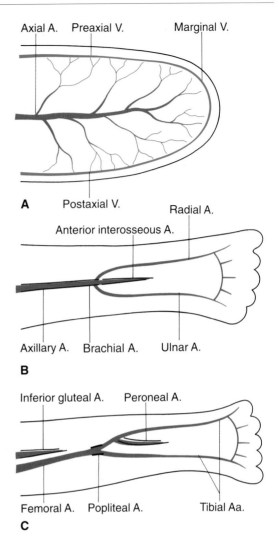

Figure 12.10. (A) Arrangement of vessels in the limb bud at 5 weeks. (B) Definitive main arteries of upper limb. (C) Definitive main arteries of lower limb. Persistent elements of axial arteries are outlined in black.

occurrence of a supernumerary finger or toe. *Lobster claw deformity* is produced by complete failure of the middle digital ray, resulting in loss of the metacarpal bone as well as the phalanges of the third finger. There is syndactyly of the other digits, in pairs (*Figure 12.11D*).

Deformities of the feet are seen in as many as 1% of newly born infants. The great

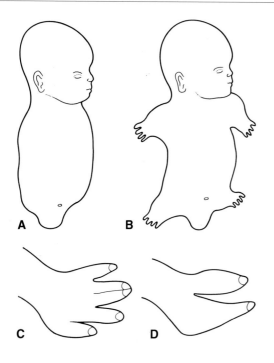

Figure 12.11. Limb malformations. (A) Amelia. (B) Meromelia. (C) Syndactyly. (D) Lobster-claw deformity.

majority are merely *postural deformations* caused by compression of the feet against the wall of the uterus for several weeks before birth; a normal shape is restored spontaneously. *Club foot* (*talipes*) is a true malformation showing a distorted posture (usually one of plantar flexion and inversion), together with skeletal malformations in the feet and some degree of muscle wasting.

The term *hip dysplasia* signifies faulty development of the hip joints. Two principal kinds of dysplasia have been identified: (a) *Capsular dysplasia* is a familial condition in which other family members experience dislocation of synovial joints because of lax ligamentous supports. *Congenital dislocation of the hip joint* may take place during delivery in this condition – especially with a 'breech' (rump-first) presentation, with the hips acutely flexed against the abdominal wall. (b) In *acetabular dysplasia*, the acetabulum faces laterally rather than downward. In consequence, the femur tends to slip out of the acetabular cup. The effect is to cause chronic hip pain during childhood and/or adolescence.

EMBRYOLOGICAL TERMS

Apical ectodermal ridge. Progress zone. Limb plates. Digital rays. Axial artery. Marginal, preaxial and postaxial veins. *Amelia. Meromelia. Syndactyly. Polydactyly. Lobster claw deformity. Club foot (talipes).*

13

Thorax: great vessels

AORTIC ARCH ARTERIES

At the end of the 4th week, the first four pairs of aortic arches pass from the aortic sac to the dorsal aorta, as described in Chapter 8. During the 5th week, the first two pairs disappear almost completely. The aortic sac also becomes Y-shaped, showing a pair of *horns* to which the third and fourth pairs of arches are attached (*Figure 13.1A*). A transient fifth pair and a prominent sixth pair are attached to the stem of the Y. The significant pairs in the human embryo are therefore numbers III, IV and VI.

INTERSEGMENTAL ARTERIES

As explained in Chapter 7, intersegmental arteries sprout from the dorsal aortas to supply the mesodermal somites and neural tube. The dorsal aortas unite from fourth thoracic to fourth lumbar somite levels, to form the descending thoracic and abdominal parts of the definitive aorta. For a time, the first eight pairs of intersegmental arteries retain their attachments to the left and right dorsal aortas above the level of fusion (*Figure 13.1A*). The seventh pair enlarge to supply the upper limb buds.

FATE OF THE THIRD ARCH ARTERIES

The third arch artery on each side forms the **stem of the internal carotid artery** (*Figure 13.1B,C*). The remainder of the internal carotid is provided by the upper end of the corresponding dorsal aorta. A sprout from the internal carotid gives rise to the **external carotid artery**.

The segment of dorsal aorta between the third and fourth arterial arches is lost on both sides. On the right, the dorsal aorta is also lost distal to the seventh intersegmental (subclavian) artery (*Figure 13.1B*).

FATE OF THE FOURTH ARCH ARTERIES

At the end of the 5th week, the heart is cranial to the upper limb buds and the dorsal aortas descend to the level of the subclavian arteries (*Figure 13.2A*). Two weeks later, the heart and limbs are at the same level, the dorsal aortas having been telescoped to accommodate the change (*Figure 13.2B*). After a further two weeks, the heart has reached its final position and the subclavian vessels *ascend* to reach the roots of the limbs (*Figure 13.2C*).

As can be seen in *Figure 13.1A–C*, the ascent of the subclavian arteries is accompanied by obliteration of the larger part of the fourth pair of aortic arches. The right one contributes to the stem of the right subclavian artery; the left contributes to the definitive aortic arch in the interval between the stems of the left common carotid and subclavian arteries.

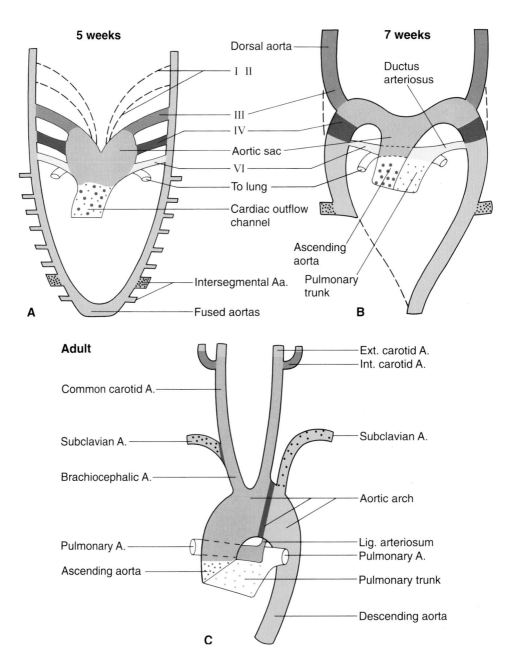

Figure 13.1. Scheme to show development of the great arteries. Roman numerals refer to embryonic arterial arches. The dashed lines in (B) represent lost segments of the dorsal aortas.

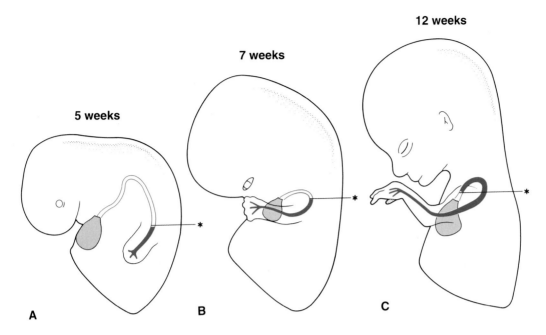

Figure 13.2. Side views showing progressive reduction of the interval between the heart and the point of origin (asterisk) of the left subclavian artery.

FATE OF THE SIXTH ARCH ARTERIES

The sixth arch arteries give offsets to the lung buds. The full lengths of the arteries proximal to the lungs become the **pulmonary arteries** (*Figure 13.3*).

On the right side, the distal portion of the sixth arch artery is lost whereas on the left, the distal portion persists throughout fetal life as the *ductus arteriosus* ('arterial duct'). The function of the arterial duct is to provide a pulmonary bypass. The fetal lungs receive only sufficient blood to establish a pulmonary vascular bed in preparation for respiratory activity; the rest is shunted to the placenta by way of the duct.

Special note: The fetal circulation, and the circulatory changes that take place after birth, are described in the final chapter of this book. A first reading of that section of the chapter is advised at this time.

FATE OF THE AORTIC SAC (*Figure 13.1A-C*)

The right horn of the aortic sac forms the **brachiocephalic artery** and the **right common carotid artery**. The left horn forms the **left common carotid artery**. The stem of the aortic sac forms the **right half of the definitive aortic arch**.

Arterial Relations of the Recurrent Laryngeal Nerves

Arrangement of the recurrent laryngeal nerves is initially symmetrical; they reach the larynx by passing beneath the sixth aortic arch arteries (*Figure 13.4A*). On the left side this relationship is preserved; the nerve eventually passes beneath the **ligamentum arteriosum** ('arterial ligament'), a fibrous remnant of the ductus arteriosus. On the right side the distal part of the sixth aortic

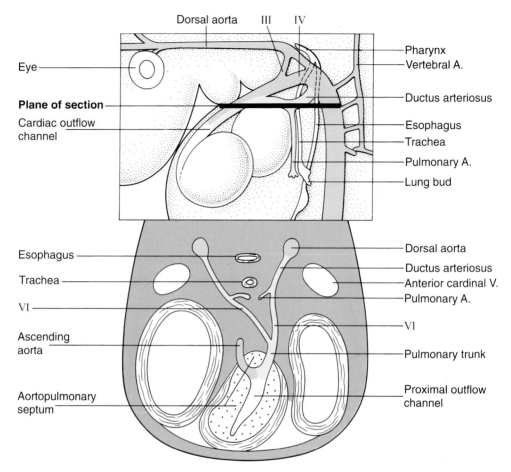

Figure 13.3. Six-week embryo in which the proximal part of the cardiac outflow channel was still undivided. (Adapted from Gasser RF, 1975, *Atlas of Human Embryos*. Hagerstown: Harper & Row.)

arch is lost, and the nerve rides up to the level of the subclavian artery (*Figure 13.4B*).

The embryonic origins of the great arteries are summarized in *Table 13.1*.

THE GREAT VEINS (*Figure 13.5*)

The **left brachiocephalic vein** diverts blood from the left to the right anterior cardinal vein. The posterior cardinal veins are almost entirely lost during the construction of the inferior vena cava, and a new, *azygos* system of veins drains the intercostal spaces.

Despite its name (Greek, *azygos*, 'unpaired'), this system is symmetrical at first. Later, however, two cross-channels convert the left azygos vein into the **hemiazygos and accessory hemiazygos veins**; both vessels drain into the **azygos vein**.

The intersegmental veins draining the upper limb buds become the **subclavian veins**, whereupon the adult pattern of the great veins is discernible. The cranial ends of the anterior cardinal veins are now the **internal jugular veins**; the **brachiocephalic veins** represent the union of internal jugular and subclavian veins; and the **upper half of the superior caval vein** is formed by the

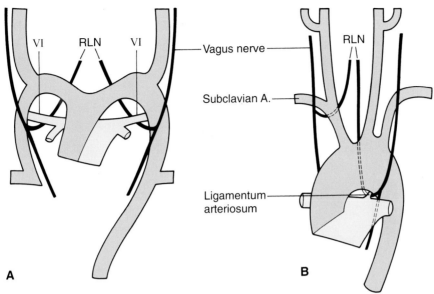

Figure 13.4. Arterial relations of the recurrent laryngeal nerves. (A) Embryonic. (B) Adult. RLN, recurrent laryngeal nerves. VI, sixth aortic arch.

Table 13.1. Embryonic origins of the great arteries

Artery	Origin
Pulmonary trunk	Truncus arteriosus
Pulmonary arteries	Sixth arch arteries
Aortic arch, right half	Aortic sac
Aortic arch, left half	Left dorsal aorta
Brachiocephalic	Aortic sac
Common carotid	Aortic sac
Proximal internal carotid	Third arch artery
Distal internal carotid	Dorsal aorta
External carotid	Sprout from third arch artery
Subclavian	Seventh intersegmental artery

Table 13.2. Embryonic origins of the great veins and of other thoracic veins

Thoracic vein	Origin
Internal jugular	Anterior cardinal
Subclavian	Seventh intersegmental
Left brachiocephalic	Left-to-right shunt vessel
Right brachiocephalic	Anterior cardinal
Superior caval vein, upper half	Anterior cardinal
Superior caval vein, lower half	Common cardinal
Arch of azygos	Right posterior cardinal
Vertical segment of azygos/hemiazygos	Azygos system
Intercostal	Thoracic intersegmental
Stem of inferior caval vein	Right hepatic
Left superior intercostal vein	Left posterior cardinal

terminal part of the anterior cardinal vein. The proximal part of the right posterior cardinal vein persists as the *arch of the azygos vein*. The right common cardinal vein becomes the **lower half of the superior caval vein**.

The left common cardinal vein becomes the **left superior intercostal vein**, draining the second and third intercostal spaces into the left brachiocephalic vein. The left

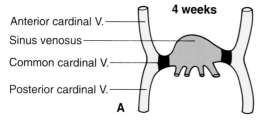

4 weeks

Anterior cardinal V.

Sinus venosus

Common cardinal V.

Posterior cardinal V.

A

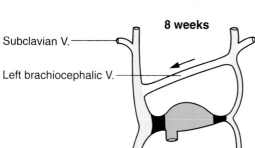

8 weeks

Subclavian V.

Left brachiocephalic V.

B

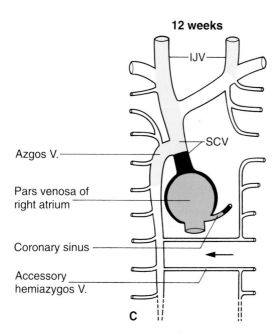

12 weeks

IJV

SCV

Azgos V.

Pars venosa of
right atrium

Coronary sinus

Accessory
hemiazygos V.

C

posterior cardinal vein gives rise only to the **oblique vein of the left atrium**, which drains into the coronary sinus.

The embryonic origins of the thoracic veins are listed in *Table 13.2.*

Figure 13.5. Scheme to show development of veins other than inferior vena cava. Note the left-to-right diversion of blood in the left brachiocephalic vein (arrow in B) and in the hemiazygos system (arrow in C). IJV, internal jugular veins; SCV, superior caval vein.

14

Thorax: the heart – early features

As noted previously in Chapter 7, the primitive heart tube originates from *cardiogenic mesoderm* in the floor of the pericardial coelom. The cranial end of the tube leads into the truncus arteriosus. The caudal end receives paired veins from the chorion and yolk sac by the end of the 3rd week, and from the embryo proper a few days later.

In the following account, positional terms from adult anatomy (e.g. anterior, above, behind) are employed where these are helpful.

PRIMITIVE HEART CHAMBERS

Figure 14.1 shows the anatomy of the heart tube at the beginning of the 4th week. The tube has a crescentic outline when viewed from the side, but it is described as 'straight' because of its profile when viewed 'face on,' i.e. from its ventral aspect. It is initially suspended within the pericardial coelom by a *dorsal mesocardium* derived from the splanchnic mesoderm (*Figure 14.1A*).

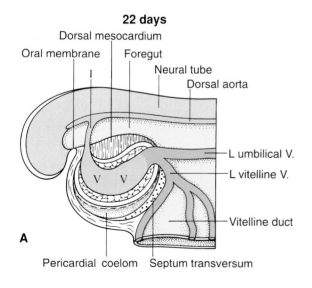

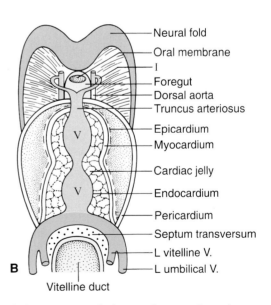

Figure 14.1. 'Straight' heart tube. (A) Viewed from the left. (B) Ventral view. I, first aortic arch; V,V, presumptive ventricles.

The wall of the heart tube comprises four layers (*Figure 14.1B*). Outermost is a delicate *epicardium*, which forms the serous pericardium lining the surface of the heart. Deep to this is the *myocardium*, which forms the contractile and conducting tissues of the heart. Innermost is the *endocardium*, a squamous endothelial cell lining continuous with that of the blood vessels. Between myocardium and endocardium is a layer of *cardiac jelly*, consisting of branched mesenchymal cells in a gelatinous matrix.

The lumen displays two dilatations, which represent the *presumptive ventricles* (specifically, the trabeculated portions of the ventricles) of the embryonic heart.

Figure 14.2 shows the internal anatomy of the heart tube at around 25 days (only the endocardium of the wall is represented). The heart tube has buckled, taking the form of a twisted U. This is the *ventricular loop*. It comprises a caudal or descending limb and a cranial or ascending limb. The caudal limb commences in a third expansion, the *common*

atrium; it leads through a *common atrioventricular canal* into the presumptive left ventricle. The cranial limb commences in the presumptive right ventricle; it leads into a long *outflow channel* connecting it to the aortic sac. The outflow channel includes the truncus arteriosus (see later).

While the ventricular loop is being formed, the mesocardium breaks down, creating the **transverse sinus** of the pericardium (*Figure 14.2A*). The transverse sinus is recognizable in the adult state as the interval between the arterial and venous perforations of the pericardial sac.

The common atrium is above and behind the primitive ventricle. It receives blood from the *sinus venosus* ('venous sinus') which is the fourth and final chamber of the embryonic heart. The sinus venosus receives the confluence of the vitelline, umbilical and common cardinal veins. It is not fully formed, nor entirely contained within the pericardial cavity, until the end of the 4th week (see below).

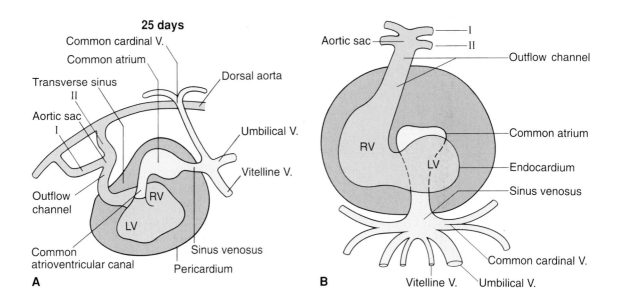

Figure 14.2. The ventricular loop. (A) Viewed from the left. (B) Ventral view. I, II, first and second aortic arches; LV, RV, presumptive left and right ventricles.

THE HEART AT 4 WEEKS

The Exterior

Figure 14.3 depicts the outward appearances of the heart at the end of the 4th week. The U shape of the ventricular loop is obvious in the side view (*Figure 14.3A*). The common atrium has expanded on each side of the outflow channel, enabling the *presumptive left and right atria* to be named (*Figure 14.3B*). Atrioventricular grooves are apparent between the atria and the ventricles, as well as an interventricular groove between the two ventricles.

The sinus venosus overlies the posterior atrioventricular groove (*Figure 14.3C*); It comprises a main part or body, together with *left and right horns*. The left horn and body empty into the right horn, and the right horn empties in turn into the right atrium through a *sinuatrial orifice*.

The left atrium receives a single *pulmonary vein* which receives tributaries from capillary plexuses surrounding the lung buds.

The Interior

Figure 14.4 represents a frontal section through the descending, proximal limb of the ventricular loop. The two halves of the common atrium are in free communication, with no sign as yet of any partition between them. The sinuatrial orifice, guarded by *left and right venous valves*, is a major feature on the posterior wall of the right atrium. The single pulmonary venous opening is a minor feature in the left atrium.

The common atrial chamber opens into the *left* ventricle through the common atrioventricular canal. Partitioning of the ventricles is commencing, with the expansion of these chambers on each side of a blunt *primary interventricular septum*. The ridges

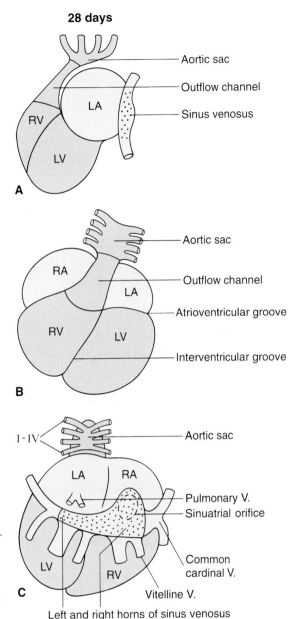

Figure 14.3. Embryonic heart at 4 weeks. (A) Left side. (B) Front. (C) Back. LA, RA, presumptive left and right atria; LV, RV, presumptive left and right ventricles.

appearing on the ventricular walls are forerunners of the **trabeculae carneae** of the adult ventricles.

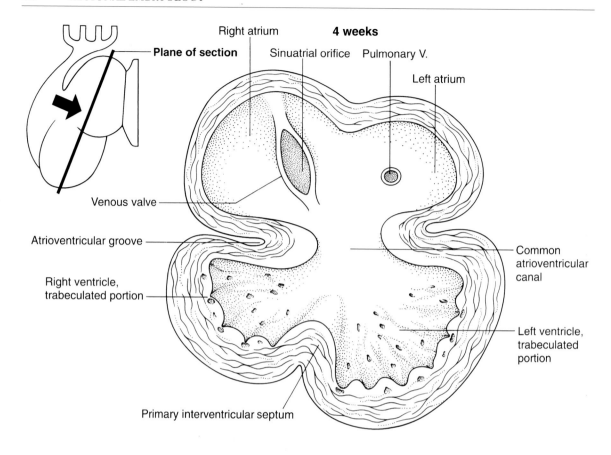

Figure 14.4. Frontal section through the descending limb of the ventricular loop.

Figure 14.5 is a frontal section through the ascending, distal limb of the ventricular loop. The trabeculated portions of the ventricles are linked to one another by a large *primary interventricular foramen*, in the interval between the interventricular septum and a ledge caused by the *primary fold* of the heart tube. The primary fold was formed by the buckling process involved in formation of the ventricular loop. The deep external groove created by the fold is continuous with the interventricular groove, thereby completing a ring around the heart that marks the position of the primary foramen.

The outflow channel of the heart begins at the level of the primary fold, and extends all the way to the aortic sac. The wall of the channel contains myocardium in its lower part, and tunica media (smooth muscle of truncus arteriosus) in its upper part.

Course of Blood Through the Heart *(Figure 14.6)*

Having entered the sinus venosus (1), the blood passes through the sinuatrial orifice into the common atrium (2). From here it passes through the common atrioventricular canal (3) into the left ventricle (4). The interventricular foramen (5) allows free passage into the right ventricle (6).

From the right ventricle, the blood passes along the outflow channel: first along the segment walled by myocardium (7a), then along the segment (truncus arteriosus) walled by smooth muscle (7b). It finally

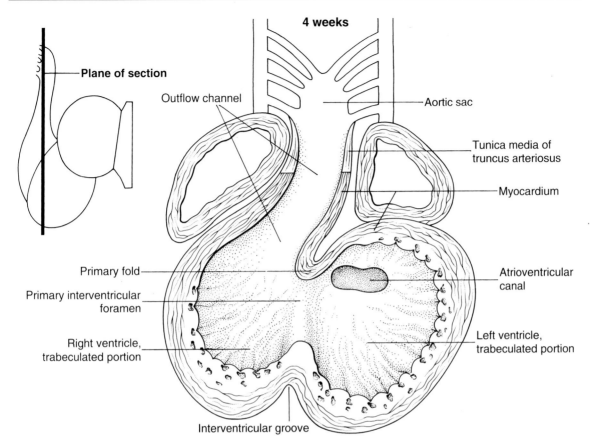

Figure 14.5. Frontal section through the ascending limb of the ventricular loop. (The outflow channel has been pulled forward.)

enters the aortic sac (8), for distribution through the four pairs of aortic arches that exist at this time.

From the above account, it is clear that the chambers of the heart at the end of the 4th week are disposed *in series*. This arrangement is sufficient to drive a single circulatory loop, from the heart to the placenta and back. By the end of the 8th week, i.e. by the end of the embryonic period, the heart will have been partitioned into two sets of chambers arranged *in parallel*. Duplication of the chambers and connecting channels is necessary for the construction of the pulmonary circulation: vascular pathways to and from

the lungs are completed during the second month, even though they have no respiratory role before birth.

Sarcomeres differentiate quickly within the muscle cells of the heart wall. Spontaneous, *myogenic* contractions begin with completion of the ventricular loop, and blood is being driven through the chorionic capillary bed a few days later. The efficiency of the newly beating heart is remarkable, given the absence of valve leaflets at the ventricular inlet and outlet. Presumably, the venous valves guarding the sinuatrial orifice are sufficient to prevent backfiring of blood during ventricular contraction.

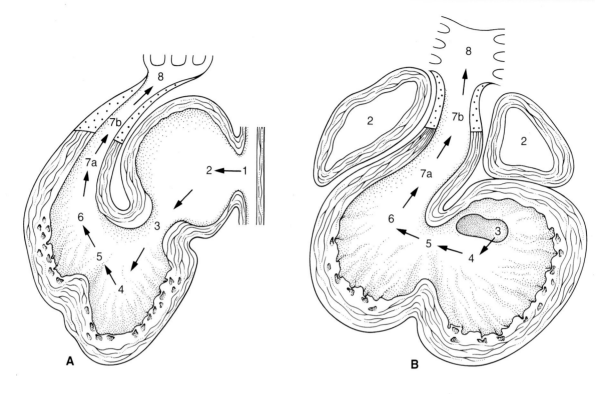

Figure 14.6. Pathway followed by the blood at 4 weeks. (A) Side view. (B) Ventral view. For the numbers, see text.

NEURAL CREST CONTRIBUTION TO THE DEVELOPING HEART

As already noted in Chapter 10, cells of the neural crest migrate widely within the embryo. They are called *mesectoderm* because they differentiate into tissues of mesodermal type such as connective tissue and cartilage, also into peripherally located nerve cells. Different genes are expressed in these cells under the influence of the various locations, with corresponding varieties of cellular phenotypes once histogenesis gets under way.

Evidence from comparative embryology (chick, rat) indicates that cells of the neural crest, originating at the level of the occipital somites, migrate to the wall of the outflow channel of the heart (*Figure 14.7*). Special

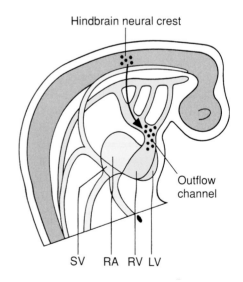

Figure 14.7. Four week heart viewed from the right. Arrow indicates migration of neural crest cells. LV, RV, left and right ventricles; RA, right atrium; SV, sinus venosus.

identification techniques indicate that neural crest cells form the tunica media of the ascending aorta and pulmonary trunk, and that they contribute connective tissue to the leaflets of the arterial valves.

EMBRYOLOGICAL TERMS

Cardiogenic mesoderm. Dorsal mesocardium. Cardiac jelly. Presumptive ventricles. Ventricular loop. Common atrium. Common atrioventricular canal. Outflow channel. Sinuatrial orifice. Presumptive atria. Venous valves. Primary interventricular septum and foramen. Primary fold.

15

Thorax: the heart – atria

PARTITIONING OF THE PRIMITIVE ATRIUM

Lateral and Frontal Views of Atrial Development

Figure 15.1 shows the internal anatomy of the common atrium at the end of the 5th week. Salient features are as follows:

- The right horn of the sinus venosus opens into the right half of the primitive atrium, the sinuatrial orifice being guarded by a pair of *venous valve*s.
- A single *primitive pulmonary vein* enters the left half of the atrium. It receives a tributary from each of the developing lungs.
- The atrioventricular (A-V) canal has been divided into left and right channels by a pair of gelatinous *subendocardial tubercles* (*endocardial cushions*).
- A crescentic *septum primum* ('first septum') has grown into the chamber from its dorsal and upper walls. The advancing edge of this thin septum fuses with the A-V endocardial cushions. In the interval between the septum and the cushions, the two halves of the primitive atrium communicate for a few days through the *foramen primum*.

Figure 15.2 presents the same two views at the end of the 7th week. The following changes have taken place:

- The right horn of the sinus venosus is being incorporated into the primitive atrium. The opening of the left horn into the right horn is visible from the interior of the atrium.
- The number of pulmonary veins has increased to two.
- The leading edge of the septum primum has fused with the A-V cushions. Communication between the two halves of the primitive atrium is being maintained through the *foramen secundum*, formed by breakdown of the cranial part of the septum primum.
- A second fold, the *septum secundum* ('second septum'), is extending into the right half of the common atrium from its roof. This is a relatively thick septum, being formed by an infolding of the atrial walls. It occupies the interval between the septum primum and the sinuatrial orifice.

Figure 15.3 shows the anatomy at the end of the 8th week, following completion of atrial partitioning. Note the following features:

- The right horn of the sinus venosus has been incorporated completely into the **right atrium**, where it forms the smooth-walled **pars venosa** ('venous component'). The left horn of the sinus venosus has become the **coronary sinus**, which drains

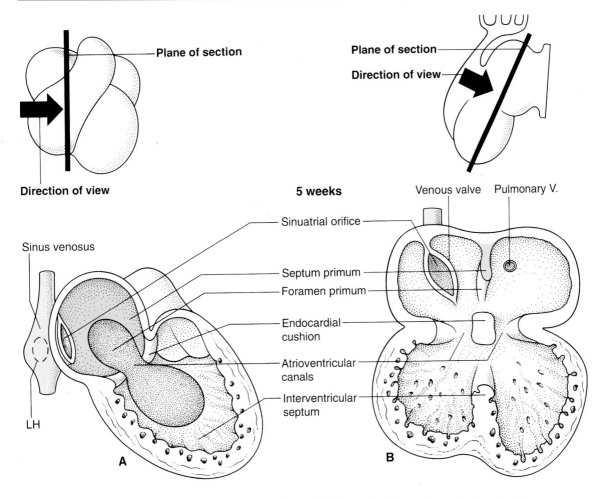

Figure 15.1. Primitive atrium at 5 weeks. (A) View of the interior from the right. In the sinus venosus, LH represents the left horn seen end-on through the right horn. (B) Ventral view of the interior.

into the pars venosa. Also entering the venous component of the right atrium are the superior caval vein, derived from the cardinal system of veins, and the inferior caval vein, derived from the vitelline system. The right venous valve guarding the sinu-atrial orifice forms the **crista terminalis**, the **valve of the inferior caval vein**, and the **valve of the coronary sinus**.

- The number of pulmonary veins has increased to four.
- The **interatrial septum** is formed by the septum primum in the floor of the oval

fossa, and by the septum secundum around it.

Together, the septum primum and septum secundum divide the primitive atrium into **right and left atria**.

Conduction System

The conduction system (conducting system) of the mature heart comprises the sinoatrial and atrioventricular nodes, together with the bundle of His and its branches on and within the ventricular walls. All of these ele-

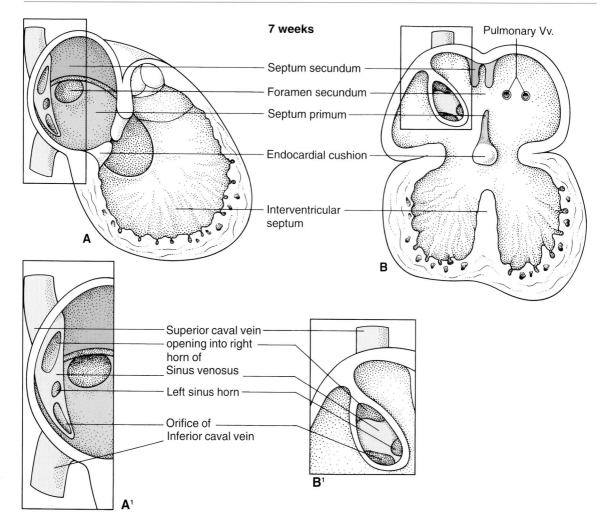

Figure 15.2. Interior of primitive atrium at 7 weeks. (A) View from the right side. (A¹) enlargement of sinuatrial orifice. (B) Ventral view. (B¹) Enlargement of sinuatrial orifice.

ments consist of modified myocardial cells.

Nodal tissue develops in the walls of the sinus venosus. Following the partial inclusion of the sinus within the right atrium, the nodal tissue condenses (a) close to the entry point of the superior caval vein, as the **sinuatrial node**; and (b) close to the right atrioventricular orifice, as the **atrioventricular node** (*Figure 15.3B¹*). The **bundle of His** develops *in situ*, and runs along the free edge of the primary interventricular septum.

Posterior Views of Atrial Development

Figure 15.4 presents posterior views of the heart at the end of the 4th, 6th and 8th weeks.

- At 4 weeks, the sinus venosus receives the paired vitelline, umbilical and common cardinal veins. A single primitive pulmonary vein opens into the left part of the common atrium.
- At 6 weeks, the left horn of the sinus is

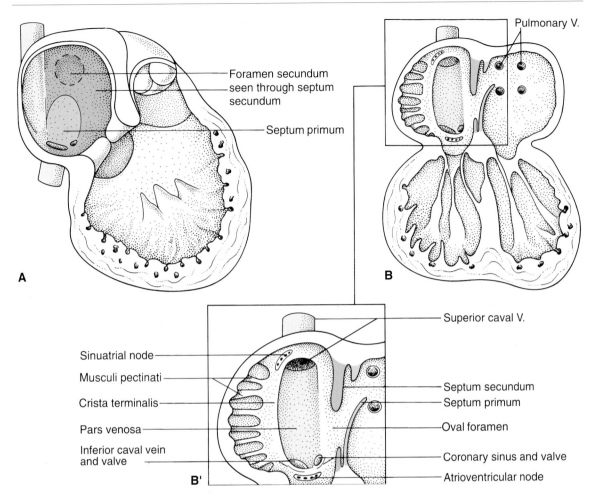

Figure 15.3. Completion of atrial partitioning. (A) View from the right side. (B) Ventral view. (B¹) Enlargement from B.

growing relatively slowly; the right horn is being incorporated into the right atrium. Two pairs of pulmonary veins open into the left atrium.

- At 8 weeks, the left horn of the sinus venosus has remained small. It persists as the **coronary sinus**, which drains most of the blood from the coronary circulation into the right atrium. *The coronary sinus is the only vein in the body containing a tunica media composed of cardiac muscle.* The right horn of the sinus venosus has formed the pars venosa of the right atrium. Most of the left atrium is formed by incorporation of pul-

monary veins, with the result that the four definitive pulmonary veins open independently into this chamber.

THE FETAL INTERATRIAL SHUNT

Deoxygenated blood from the fetal circulation is returned to the right atrium by way of the superior caval vein (*Figure 15.5*). This blood passes through the tricuspid valve into the right ventricle. Oxygenated blood from the placenta enters the right atrium by way

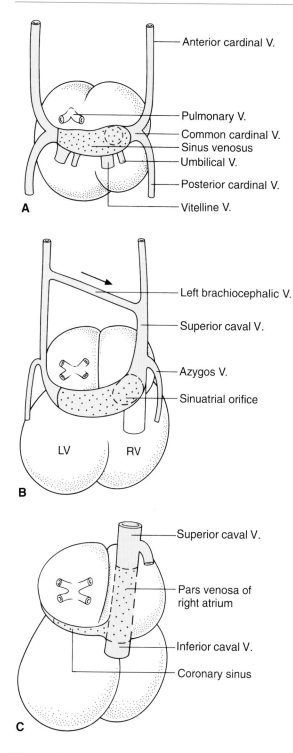

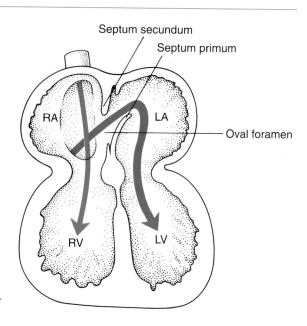

Figure 15.5. Intracardiac portion of the fetal circulation. Oxygenated blood entering from the placenta via the inferior caval vein is shown in red. Deoxygenated blood returning from the upper half of the body via the superior caval vein is blue. RA, LA, right and left atria; RV, LV, right and left ventricles.

of the inferior caval vein. This blood passes through the *oval foramen* into the left atrium. The oval foramen is bounded by the septum secundum, and the thin septum primum acts as a flap valve, preventing reflux from the right atrium. The function of the oval foramen is to allow the oxygenated blood to bypass the nonfunctioning lungs. From the left atrium, the blood flows through the bicuspid (mitral) valve into the left ventricle.

POSTNATAL APPEARANCE OF THE RIGHT ATRIUM (*Figure 15.6*)

After birth, the oval foramen is sealed off by the septum primum. Thereafter, the septum primum forms the floor of the **oval fossa**

Figure 15.4. Dorsal views of sinus venosus (stippled). (A) At 4 weeks. (B) At 6 weeks. (C) At 8 weeks. LV, RV, left and right ventricles.

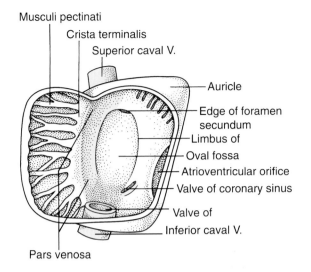

Musculi pectinati
Crista terminalis
Superior caval V.
Auricle
Edge of foramen secundum
Limbus of
Oval fossa
Atrioventricular orifice
Valve of coronary sinus
Valve of
Inferior caval V.
Pars venosa

Figure 15.6. Interior of right atrium a week after birth.

(fossa ovalis) whose margin (**limbus**) represents the edge of the septum secundum.

The smooth-walled **pars venosa** (venous component of right atrium) is derived from the right horn of the sinus venosus. The rough-walled anterior portion of the atrium, including the **auricle** (appendage), is derived from the right half of the primitive atrium.

POSTNATAL APPEARANCE OF THE LEFT ATRIUM

The main part of the left atrium is smooth-walled and is derived from incorporation of pulmonary veins. Only the rough-walled left auricle originates from the primitive atrium.

SUMMARY

The embryonic origins of the atria and related veins are summarized in Table 15.1.

Table 15.1 Embryonic origins of the atria and related veins

Heart chamber/vein	Embryonic origin
Coronary sinus	Sinus venosus, left horn
Oblique vein of left atrium	Left common cardinal vein
Right atrium, pars venosa	Sinus venosus, right horn
Right atrium, trabeculated part including auricle	Primitive atrium
Crista terminalis, valves of inferior vena cava and of coronary sinus	Right sinuatrial valve
Left atrium, smooth-walled part	Primitive pulmonary veins
Left auricle	Primitive atrium

EMBRYOLOGICAL TERMS

Venous valves. Primitive pulmonary vein. Subendocardial tubercles (endocardial cushions). Septum primum. Foramen primum. Foramen secundum. Septum secundum. Oval foramen. Pars venosa (venous component) of right atrium.

16

Thorax: the heart – ventricles and outflow channels

CHAPTER SUMMARY

Partitioning of the ventricles and outflow channel
  Early partitioning
  Completion of the outflow partition
  Closure of the interventricular foramen
  Development of the valves
Outflow channels in the mature heart

During weeks 5 and 6, the ventricles and the outflow channel are transformed from a single, in-series pathway into the double pathway characteristic of the mature heart.

PARTITIONING OF THE VENTRICLES AND OUTFLOW CHANNEL

Early Partitioning

At the end of the 4th week, the outflow channel of the heart connects the right ventricle to the aortic sac (refer to *Figure 14.5*). The proximal part of the channel is surrounded by myocardium, the distal part by the mesenchyme of the truncus arteriosus, formed in large part by cells derived from the neural crest (Chapter 14).

Events taking place at the commencement of the 5th week are depicted in *Figure 16.1*. The *aortopulmonary septum* makes its first appearance in the root of the truncus, projecting into the lumen from the dorsal wall. The sixth pair of aortic arches have just appeared, and they open into the truncus on the left side of the septum. It is then possible to define a *pulmonary orifice* of the heart mainly to the left of the septum, and an *aortic orifice* mainly to the right.

The aortopulmonary septum extends proximally in the form of two *ridges*, composed initially of endocardial cushion tissue. The arrows in *Figure 16.1* indicate the migration of neural crest cells into the ridges, from the root of the truncus arteriosus. These cells have the property of inducing migration of myocardial cells into the cushions. The outcome is that the septum becomes muscular, except for the short segment retained in the root of the truncus.

Figure 16.2 represents a ventral (front) view of the heart half way through the 5th week. For this figure and the next, the outflow channel and the trabeculated parts of the ventricles will be described separately.

Outflow Channel

The two aortopulmonary ridges are extending proximally. The *right-anterior* ridge descends obliquely across the anterior wall of the outflow channel, to end on the right side of the channel. The *left-posterior* ridge descends along the posterior wall, toward the primary fold.

Trabeculated Parts of Ventricles

The interventricular groove on the outer surface of the heart is matched internally by

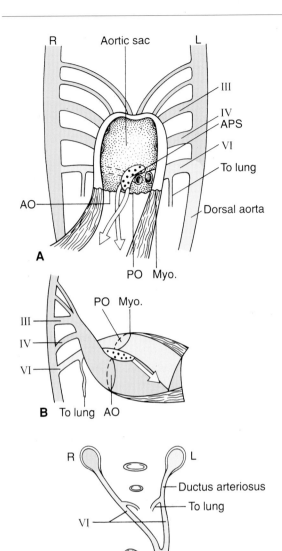

A

B To lung AO

C

Figure 16.1. First appearance of the aortopulmonary septum (APS). Roman numerals indicate aortic arches. Arrows indicate migrations of neural crest cells. AO, PO, aortic and pulmonary orifices (future sites of semilunar valves); Myo, distal limit of myocardium in the outflow channel. (A) Ventral view. (B) Right side. (C) Transverse section.

the interventricular septum, which is created by myocardial infolding along the groove. The free edge of the septum contains myocardial cells which will become conduction tissue (conducting tissue) later on. Fortunately, the ring of conduction tissue is histochemically distinctive from the outset, thereby enabling its remarkable history to be followed during the completion of partitioning. In what follows, it is referred to as the *ventricular ring*.

The common atrioventricular canal is beginning to expand transversely, moving the posterior part of the ventricular ring a little to the right. (The anterior part of the ring has been left in place in this and later illustrations, although it belongs to the anterior wall of the heart.) Note that all of the blood must pass through the ring, on its way from the left to the right ventricle.

Figure 16.3 (p.99) illustrates the interior at the end of the 5th week. The following changes have taken place:

- *Outflow channels.* The free margins of the aortopulmonary ridges are fusing, to divide the outflow channel. An anterior, *pulmonary* channel passes initially in front of the septum and ends to the left of the septum at the level of the sixth aortic arches. The posterior, *aortic* channel passes behind the septum and ends to its right, at the level of the aortic sac (from which the third and fourth pairs of aortic arches originate).
- *Trabeculated parts of ventricles.* The ventricular chambers are enlarging, thereby increasing the height of the interventricular septum. The superior and inferior atrioventricular endocardial cushions have fused, forming a seam across the posterior wall of the interventricular foramen. Now, for the first time, the right atrium is opening into the right ventricle, providing direct access to the outflow channel. The

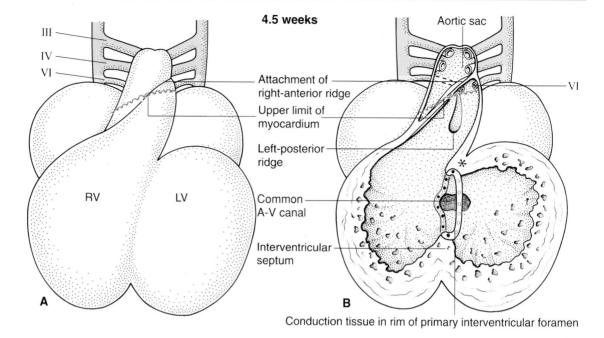

Figure 16.2. Ventricles and outflow channels. (A) Ventral view. RV, LV, right and left ventricles. (B) Same, with ventral wall removed except for anterior rim of primary interventricular foramen. Asterisk above ventricular ring marks the primary fold.

left atrioventricular canal has been displaced to the left by the fused cushion tissue; access to the outflow channel is posterior to the apex of the primary fold and the left part of the aortopulmonary septum.

The ventricular ring now has three parts. One part remains along the anterior and inferior edges of the interventricular foramen. A second part passes around the right atrioventricular canal. A third part almost completely encircles the future outflow channel from the left ventricle.

Completion of the Outflow Partition

A photograph of the heart of a 6-week embryo is shown in *Figure 16.4*. Of particular interest is the X-shaped configuration of the outflow channels, which are lodged in a deep groove between the two atria. The lower end of the aortic channel has obliterated the upper end of the interventricular groove, having incorporated the primary fold.

The interior of such a specimen is shown in *Figure 16.5*. Significant advances have taken place during the 6th week:

- Division of the outflow channel has been completed.
- Aortic and pulmonary valves mark the junction of the divided channel with the truncus arteriosus.
- The posterior wall of the pulmonary outflow channel extends from the pulmonary valve to the **supraventricular crest**, a muscular ridge marking the proximal end of the aortopulmonary septum. The anterior wall extends proximally to the level of the **septomarginal trabecula**, a muscular ridge passing from the interventricular

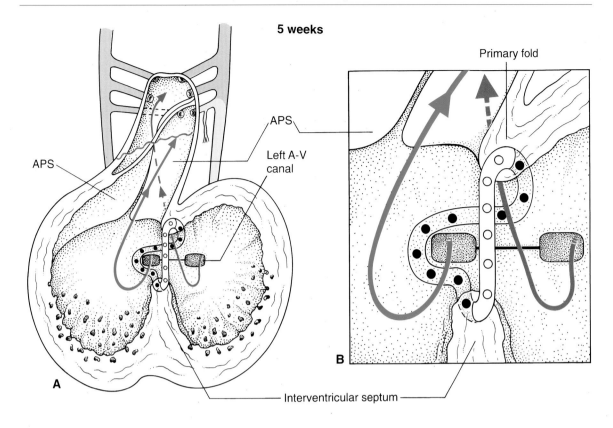

5 weeks

Primary fold

APS

APS

Left A-V
canal

APS

Interventricular septum

Figure 16.3. Interior of ventricles and outflow channels prior to completion of aortopulmonary septum (APS). (B) Enlargement from (A). Arrows indicate the course taken by the two blood streams.

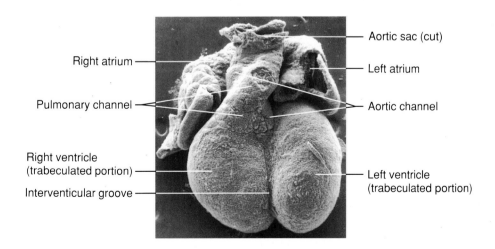

Right atrium

Aortic sac (cut)

Left atrium

Pulmonary channel

Aortic channel

Right ventricle
(trabeculated portion)

Interventicular groove

Left ventricle
(trabeculated portion)

Figure 16.4. Scanning electron micrograph of the heart at 6 weeks; ventral view. (Photograph kindly provided by Professor S. Viragh, Postgraduate Medical School, Budapest.)

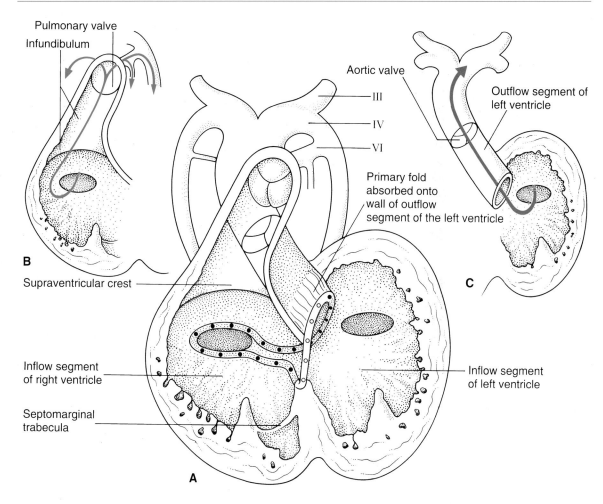

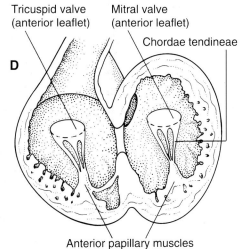

Figure 16.5. Ventricles and outflow channels at 6 weeks. (A) Ventral view of interior; dashed lines indicate aortic channel behind the infundibulum. (B) Pulmonary channel. (C) Aortic channel. (D) Atrioventricular valves.

septum to the **anterior papillary muscle** of the right ventricle. It is now possible to describe the right ventricle as comprising an *inflow segment* extending from the atrioventricular orifice to the large oval marked off by the two muscular ridges just described; and an *outflow segment* extending from the level of the oval, all the way to the pulmonary valve. The trabeculated part of the ventricle contributes to the inlet segment, and to the anterior wall of the outflow segment. The funnel-shaped part of the outflow segment, extending distally from the supraventricular crest, is the smooth-walled **infundibulum**. The course taken by the blood entering from the right atrium is shown in *Figure 16.5B*.

- The aortic outflow channel has moved further to the left, having incorporated the primary fold. The proximal end of the channel is close to the left atrioventricular canal. The left ventricle can now be described as comprising an *inflow segment*, commencing at the left atrioventricular opening and including the entire trabeculated part; and a smooth-walled *outflow segment* extending distally, to the aortic valve. The outflow segment is the future **aortic vestibule**.

- The course taken by blood entering from the left atrium is shown in *Figure 16.5C*.

Closure of the Interventricular Foramen

Figure 16.6 shows the right side of the primary interventricular septum, toward the end of the embryonic period. The interventricular foramen occupies the upper, posterior corner of the septum. The conduction tissue present beneath the foramen initially formed the lower half of the ventricular ring. It is the only part of the rim that survives to a significant extent. It is connected to the atrioventricular node, and it enlarges to become the **bundle of His**. At the anterior margin of the foramen the main bundle divides into right and left bundle branches, which descend on the respective sides of the interventricular septum. The right bundle branch runs mainly to the anterior papillary muscle, within the septomarginal trabecula.

The tissue closing the interventricular foramen forms the membranous part of the interventricular septum, which is devoid of muscle. Together with the other, muscular

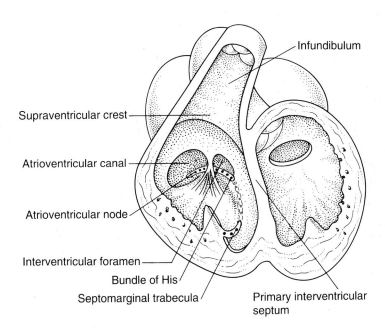

Figure 16.6. Interventricular foramen just prior to closure. The atrioventricular valves are not shown.

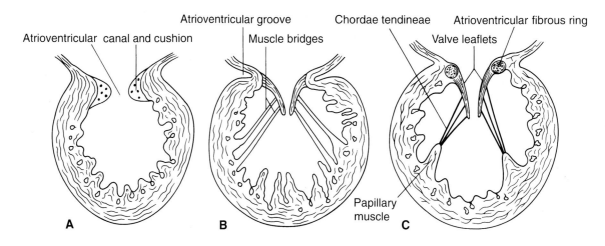

Figure 16.7. Scheme showing development of the atrioventricular valves.

part, it completes the secondary or **definitive interventricular septum**. The precise mechanism of closure of the foramen is not understood as yet, although it is of particular interest because a septal defect in this region is the single most common malformation of the heart. Potential contributors include the adjacent edge of the primary septum, the left-posterior aortopulmonary ridge, and the cushion tissue that divided the common atrioventricular canal.

Development of the Valves

The valves of the heart develop initially from the endocardial cushion tissue located in the atrioventricular canals and in the distal part of the outflow channel. Development begins during the 5th week, and is complete by the end of the embryonic period.

Atrioventricular Valves

Each atrioventricular canal contains a remnant of the cushion tissue that divided the common canal in two (*Figure 16.7*). The cushion tissue is invaded by mesenchyme, which projects into the lumen of the canal.

Three projections are found in the case of the **tricuspid (right atrioventricular) valve**, and two for the **bicuspid (mitral) valve**. At the same time, the inner walls of the ventricles are being excavated (*Figure 16.8*). Some of the excavations form **trabeculae carneae**, and some form bridges of muscle connected to the outer (mural) surfaces of the mesenchymal projections. Partial replacement of the bridges by collagenous tissue yields **papillary muscles** and **chordae tendineae**. The mesenchymal projections also become fibrous, yielding the **leaflets** of the valves. A further condensation of mesenchyme, along the lines of mural attachment of the leaflets, gives rise to the **atrioventricular fibrous rings**.

Semilunar Valves

The pulmonary and aortic semilunar valves develop along the distal edge of the myocardium in the outflow tract (*Figure 16.9A*). Cushion tissue lines the inner wall of the tract, and, along the line of fusion of the aortopulmonary ridges, two pairs of valvar tubercles appear (*Figure 16.9B*). A further tubercle appears on the opposite wall on each side, yielding a total of three for the

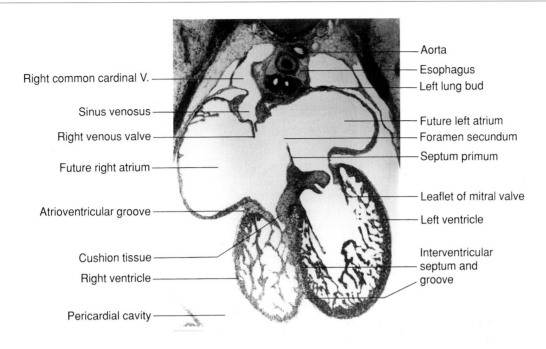

Figure 16.8. Frontal section through the heart at 7 weeks. (University of Washington Collection.)

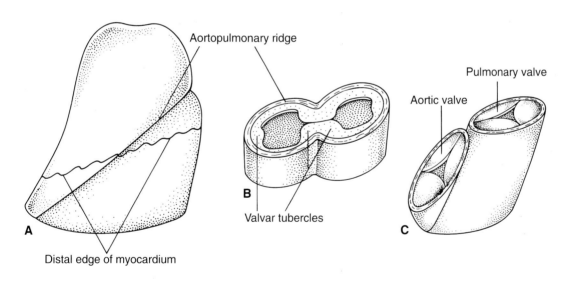

Figure 16.9. Development of the semilunar valves. (A) Outflow channel from Fig. 16.2. (B) Transverse section along edge of myocardium. (C) Later stage.

infundibulum and three for the aortic vestibule. All of the tubercles are invaded by mesenchyme containing neural crest cells, and become converted into the leaflets of the **pulmonary and aortic valves** (*Figure 16.9C*). Increasing obliquity of the aortic channel causes the aortic valve to face away from the pulmonary valve.

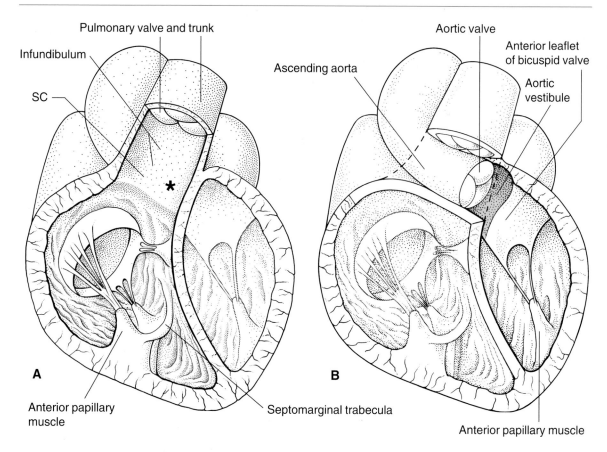

Figure 16.10. Ventricles in the mature heart. (A) Right ventricle; asterisk indicates portion of infundibulum related to the aortic vestibule. SC, supraventricular crest. (B) Left ventricle. Aortic vestibule is shown in red. Dashed lines indicate position of the infundibulum.

OUTFLOW CHANNELS IN THE MATURE HEART

The outflow channels of the mature heart are illustrated in *Figure 16.10*. The *right* ventricular outflow channel comprises the trabeculated ventricle in front of the septomarginal trabecula, and the infundibulum leading from the supraventricular crest to the pulmonary valve. The **pulmonary trunk** has developed from the truncus arteriosus. The *left* ventricular outflow channel undergoes a relative shrinkage during fetal life, associated with replacement of myocardial cells by fibrous tissue. In the mature heart, the ventricular outflow channel reaches from the line of attachment of the anterior leaflet of the bicuspid valve to the left atrioventricular fibrous ring, to the scalloped line of attachment of the leaflets of the aortic valve to the aortic orifice of the heart – a distance of about 1 cm. The reduction of the aortic vestibule is accompanied by elongation of the root of the aorta, such that **ascending aorta** replaces aortic vestibule behind the infundibulum, except at its lower end.

17

Thorax: cardiovascular malformations

MALFORMATIONS OF THE HEART

Congenital malformations of the heart are the most frequent group of serious malformations, with an incidence of around 8 per 1000 live births. In the case of stillbirths and spontaneous abortions, the incidence seems to be as great as 10%. Most cardiovascular malformations have no identifiable cause, and are regarded as multifactorial, i.e. produced by a genetic predisposition acting in concert with unknown environmental influences. About 10% of live-born infants with congenital heart disease have chromosomal abnormalities, such as trisomy 21 (Down's syndrome), trisomy 18, trisomy 13, or Turner's syndrome (monosomy X). Identified environmental causes include rubella (German measles), anticonvulsant drugs and heavy alcohol intake. The most vulnerable period of cardiovascular development is the 3rd through the 7th week.

Cardiovascular malformations are potentially dangerous in two ways. First, they may produce arteriovenous shunts which put the circulation at a mechanical disadvantage. In some cases so much blood bypasses the lungs that the infant is cyanotic even at rest (so-called 'blue baby'). Secondly, one or more of the heart channels may be so narrowed as to cause congestive heart failure in childhood, or to render mechanically stressed areas of the endocardium susceptible to blood-borne disease; for example, bacterial endocarditis may result from dental or tonsillar infections.

Anatomical varieties of cardiovascular malformations, occurring alone or in combination, number more than one hundred. The following list accounts for about 80% of cases: atrial or atrioventricular septal defect; ventricular septal defect; pulmonary or aortic stenosis; Fallot's tetralogy; persistent ductus arteriosus; and coarctation of the aorta. Less frequent defects to be mentioned are: transposition of the great arteries; common arterial trunk; double inlet left ventricle; and anomalies of position and disposition of the heart.

Atrial and Atrioventricular Septal Defects

An isolated atrial septal defect almost always takes the form of a defect in the oval fossa (*Figure 17.1A*). The fault lies in an unduly large foramen secundum (within the septum primum), permitting a significant left-to-right shunt of oxygenated blood, with recirculation through the lungs. Conventionally, this defect is referred to as an *ostium secundum lesion*. It should be pointed out that a small defect, known as 'probe patency,' occurs in 25% of the population and is without significance.

Less frequent is an *atrioventricular septal defect*, also known as *common atrioventricular canal*. This is the most frequent defect found in children with Down's syndrome. The anatomy (*Figure 17.1B*) comprises a low atrial septal defect, a single atrioventricular canal bridged by a valve attached to both ventricular walls, and a ventricular inlet septal defect. The core of the heart may be described as 'unsprung,' i.e. to have come apart, in this condition. Normally, the core consists of the figure-of-eight fibrous skeleton formed by the atrioventricular rings. The atrioventricular endocardial cushions may provide the requisite matrix for the construction of the rings. In that sense the cushion tissue may be at fault here. Consequent shallowness of the atrioventric-

ular grooves accounts for the single, distorted valve. Where the atrioventricular valve leaflets are attached to the crest of the interventricular septum, the defect is referred to as an *ostium primum lesion*.

Ventricular Septal Defects

A defective interventricular septum is found in some 30% of malformed hearts, both in stillborn and live-born infants. The defect may occur either alone or in association with other defects. Most commonly, there is a 'perimembranous' foramen that includes the region normally sealed off by the membranous part of the interventricular septum (*Figure 17.2*). Instead, one or more perforations may be found in the muscular part of the septum. In either case, the result is a left-to-right shunt, with recirculation of oxygenated blood through the lungs.

Isolated Pulmonary Stenosis

Stenosis (narrowing) of the pulmonary trunk and/or of the pulmonary arteries most

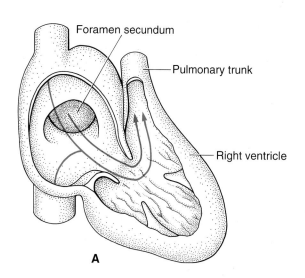
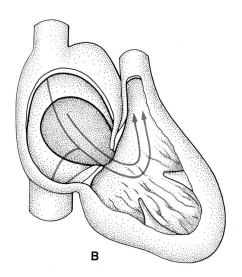

Figure 17.1. (A) Ostium secundum lesion. (B) Ostium primum lesion.

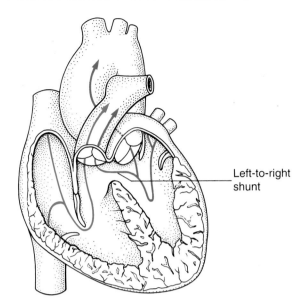

Figure 17.2. Ventricular septal defect.

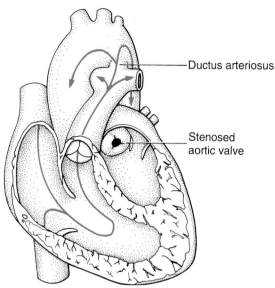

Figure 17.3. Aortic stenosis.

often follows infection with the rubella virus during the first trimester of pregnancy. The pathology is characterized by defective development of elastic tissue in the arterial walls.

Aortic Stenosis

Narrowing of the aortic channel may occur at the level of the ventricular outlet ('subaortic stenosis'), at the level of the aortic valve ('valvar atresia'), or within the aorta itself ('hypoplastic aorta'). The second two are associated with an abnormally small left ventricle, under the title 'hypoplastic left heart syndrome.' Aortic obstruction may be so severe that the systemic circuit depends upon an input from the right ventricle, through the ductus arteriosus (*Figure 17.3*).

Fallot's Tetralogy

The tetralogy of Fallot is the commonest cause of a 'blue baby.' The source of the

cyanosis is a right-to-left shunt, whereby deoxygenated blood from the right ventricle enters the aorta. The components of the tetralogy (*Figure 17.4*) are: valvar or subvalvar stenosis of the pulmonary outlet; rightward positioning of the aorta which straddles the interventricular septum; right

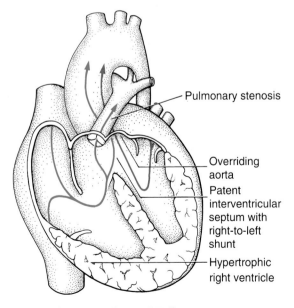

Figure 17.4. Tetralogy of Fallot.

ventricular hypertrophy; and a ventricular septal defect involving the lower end of the infundibulum.

The tetralogy has a single basis of explanation in an aortopulmonary septum that is laid down too near the front and right of the cardiac outflow channel. In consequence, the pulmonary channel is unduly narrow, leading to hyperplasia of the right ventricle as a result of back-pressure; and the aorta is unduly large and overrides a normally placed interventricular septum. The malalignment of the two septa accounts for the ventricular septal defect.

Transposition of the Great Arteries

In this condition the pulmonary trunk arises from the left ventricle and the aorta arises from the right ventricle (*Figure 17.5*). The anatomy is explained on the basis of a 'straight' aortopulmonary septum (i.e. without the normal twist). The condition is incompatible with postnatal survival unless shunting is allowed by the presence of an atrial or ventricular septal defect.

Common Arterial Trunk

Common arterial trunk is a rare defect where, at least to all appearances, an aortopulmonary septum was never laid down. A single arterial canal straddles the interventricular septum and gives rise to the coronary and pulmonary arteries and aortic arch (*Figure 17.6*).

MALFORMATIONS OF THE GREAT ARTERIES

Persistent Ductus Arteriosus

Failure of the ductus arteriosus to close after birth accounts for 10% of cardiovascular malformations present in infancy. Normally, the ductus undergoes functional closure within a few days after birth, and anatomical closure within a few weeks.

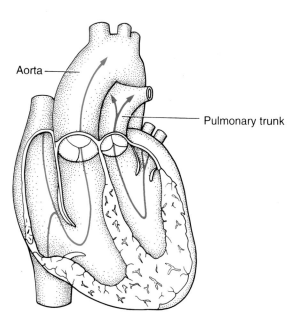

Figure 17.5. Transposition of great arteries.

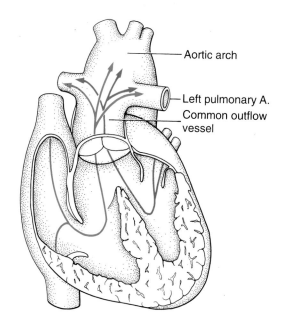

Figure 17.6. Common arterial trunk.

There is a statistical association of persistence of the duct with premature birth, where the changes preparing the duct for closure during the final few weeks of intrauterine life are forestalled.

Persistent ductus arteriosus usually occurs in isolation, but other malformations may encourage persistence by lowering the pulmonary arterial pressure – pulmonary stenosis, for example (*Figure 17.7*).

Coarctation of the Aorta

Coarctation ('choking') is manifested by narrowing of the aorta, either in the form of hypoplasia of the aortic arch as far as the level of entry of the ductus arteriosus, or in the form of a shelf projecting into the lumen of the aorta – usually proximal to the duct ('preductal coarctation,' *Figure 17.8*).

Coarctation accounts for 10% of major cardiovascular malformations. About half

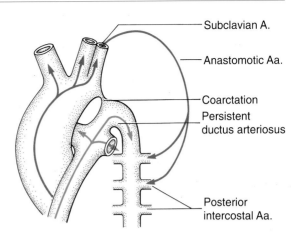

Figure 17.8. Preductal coarctation of the aorta.

have an accompanying ventricular septal defect.

Coarctation is of general medical interest in that it may remain unidentified until early adulthood. It should always be suspected in young adults presenting with high blood pressure. Physical diagnosis is simple enough if the condition is borne in mind. First, the femoral pulses are absent or reduced because propagation of the pulse wave is blocked at the level of the obstruction. Secondly, distribution of blood to the lower part of the body in these patients is by way of branches of the two subclavian arteries. (a) Blood is carried to the descending aorta via the scapular anastomosis, which connects with intercostal arteries. Wormlike wriggling of the scapular arteries may be observed through the skin and provides an obvious clue. (b) Blood is carried to the femoral arteries via the internal thoracic–superior epigastric–inferior epigastric arterial chain. Zooming of blood through the epigastric anastomosis can be heard with a stethoscope – it cannot be seen because the anastomosis runs behind the rectus abdominis muscle.

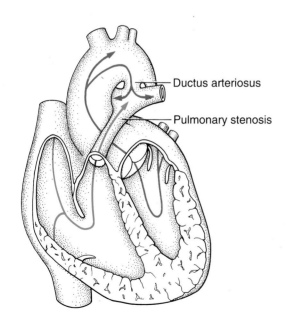

Figure 17.7. Persistent ductus arteriosus in the presence of pulmonary stenosis.

ABNORMALITIES OF POSITION AND OF DISPOSITION OF THE HEART

The briefest references will be made because the following conditions are very rare.

Ectopia cordis is a condition where the heart is completely extruded through a cleft sternum onto the body surface. Some cases can be explained by the presence of amniotic bands causing herniation of abdominal contents into the thorax.

Dextrocardia describes the state where the apex of the heart is on the right hand side, in the absence of displacement by a lesion such as diaphragmatic hernia. Arrangement of other organs is variable. (a) All of the thoracic and abdominal structures, including the heart chambers, may be a mirror image of the normal; this is *situs inversus totalis*, and the individual may be perfectly healthy. (b) The thoracic organs alone may have a mirror image arrangement, with two lobes in the right lung and three in the left; the heart is malformed in some cases, normal (except for reversed chambers) in others. (c) A state of *isomerism* ('matching') may exist, both lungs having either two lobes or three. Multiple malformations are the rule, in the heart and elsewhere.

Isolated levocardia is the state where the organs in general have a reversed arrangement but the cardiac apex is on the left side. The heart is malformed in such cases.

MALFORMATIONS OF THORACIC ARTERIES AND VEINS

Rare malformations of great arteries are shown in *Figure 17.9*. In *right-sided aortic arch* (*Figure 17.9A*), the the right dorsal aorta has been completely preserved instead of the left one. In *double aortic arch* (*Figure 17.9B*), both

Embryo   **Adult**

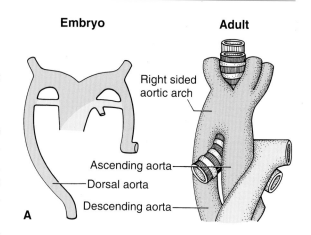

Right sided aortic arch

Ascending aorta

Dorsal aorta

Descending aorta

A

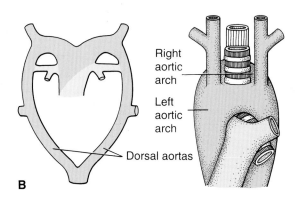

Right aortic arch

Left aortic arch

Dorsal aortas

B

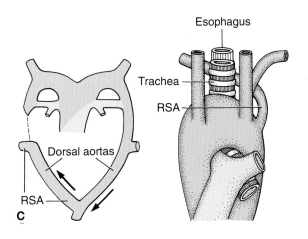

Esophagus

Trachea

RSA

Dorsal aortas

RSA

C

Figure 17.9. Malformations of great arteries. (A) Right-sided aorta. (B) Double aortic arch. (C) Anomalous origin of right subclavian artery (RSA).

dorsal aortas have been preserved. In *anomalous origin of the right subclavian artery (Figure 17.9C)*, this artery pursues an anomalous course, behind the esophagus. The latter two anomalies may cause compression of the esophagus.

Persistent left superior caval vein seems less unusual than any other anomaly described in this section – perhaps because it is easy to identify in routine chest radiographs. In some cases it is the only caval vein present (*Figure 17.10A*). In others, both caval veins are present but the left brachiocephalic vein is missing (*Figure 17.10B*). Because it is derived from the left anterior and common cardinal veins, the anomalous vein drains into the left horn of the sinus venosus, represented by the coronary sinus.

Anomalous pulmonary venous drainage results from partial or total failure of the embryonic pulmonary vascular plexuses to drain into the left atrium. Some or all of the blood is returned instead to the right atrium, through connections with one or more of the great veins.

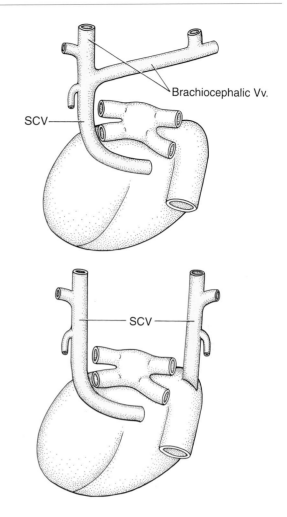

Figure 17.10. (A) Left superior caval vein (SCV). (B) Double superior caval vein (SCV).

EMBRYOLOGICAL TERMS

Ostium secundum lesion. Atrioventricular septal defect (common atrioventricular canal). Ostium primum lesion. Ventricular septal defects. Isolated pulmonary stenosis. Aortic stenosis. Fallot's tetralogy. Transposition of the great vessels. Common arterial trunk. Persistent ductus arteriosus. Coarctation of the aorta. Ectopia cordis.

Dextrocardia. Isolated levocardia. Right-sided aortic arch. Double aortic arch. Anomalous origin of right subclavian artery. Persistent left superior caval vein. Anomalous pulmonary venous drainage.

18

Thorax: lower respiratory tract, esophagus and diaphragm

LOWER RESPIRATORY TRACT

The lower respiratory tract comprises the larynx, trachea, bronchi, bronchioles and pulmonary alveoli. The entire tract develops as an outgrowth from the caudal part of the foregut.

Development of the Laryngotracheal Tube

A *laryngotracheal groove* appears in the floor of the foregut in the middle of the 4th week (*Figure 18.1*). The epithelium lining the groove contributes to the lower respiratory tract in an orderly manner (*Figure 18.2A*): the rostral part lines the **larynx**; the middle part lines the **trachea**; and the caudal part lines the **bronchial tree**. The caudal part shows an early bulge, the *respiratory diverticulum* (*Figure 18.2B*) which splits to form two *lung buds* (*Figure 18.2C*).

A septum grows into the lumen of the foregut from each side, converting the laryngotracheal groove into a *laryngotracheal tube* opening into the caudal part of the

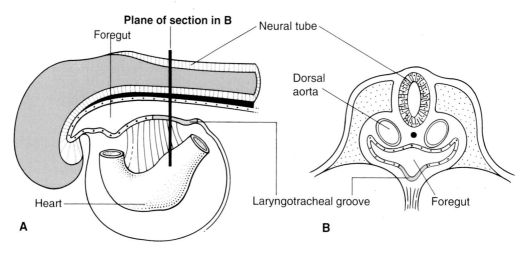

Figure 18.1. Primordium of lower respiratory tract (blue) at 24 days.

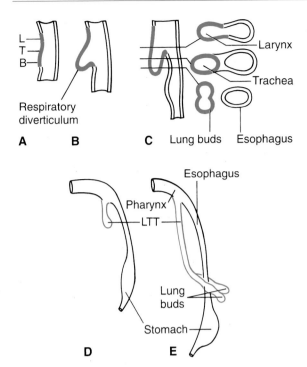

Figure 18.2. Early development of lower respiratory tract. (A) At 24 days (from *Figure 18.1*). L, T, B, presumptive epithelial linings of larynx, trachea, bronchial tree. (B) At 25 days. (C) At 26 days. (D) At 4 weeks. (E) At 5 weeks. LTT, laryngotracheal tube.

pharynx (*Figure 18.2D*). The section of foregut in the interval between the laryngeal opening and the stomach is the **esophagus** (*Figure 18.2E*).

Development of the Lungs and Pleura

The lung buds invaginate the pericardioperitoneal canals during the 5th and 6th weeks. When invaginated by the lungs, the canals become the **pleural cavities**. The invaginated coelomic epithelium covering the lungs forms the **visceral pleura**; the epithelium remaining on the walls forms the **parietal pleura**.

The connection of each pleural cavity with the pericardial cavity is reduced by a *pleuropericardial fold* containing the common cardinal vein and phrenic nerve (*Figure 18.3*). The connection with the peritoneal coelom is reduced by the *pleuroperitoneal membrane*, a sickle-shaped fold of somatic mesoderm at the level of the septum transversum.

Closure of the Pleural Cavity

With the descent of the heart into the thorax, the pleuropericardial folds become more vertical, and they fuse with the splanchnic mesoderm on the ventral aspect of the esophagus (*Figure 18.4A,B*). In this way, the pleuropericardial connection is severed.

The septum transversum and pleuroperitoneal membranes descend along with the heart, thereby lengthening the pleural cavities. Descent of the lungs and heart is arrested during the 7th week by enlargement of the liver and suprarenal glands within the abdomen (*Figure 18.5*) The pleuroperitoneal openings are sealed off by fusion of the membranes with the septum transversum.

Formation of the Fibrous Pericardium

The pleural cavities are enlarged by extension of the pleural cavities into the somatic mesoderm of the lateral and ventral abdominal wall (arrows in *Figures 18.4* and *18.5*). The somatic mesoderm peeled off in this way forms the **fibrous pericardium** enclosing the heart.

Blood Supply of the Lungs (Figure 18.5)

The developing lungs tap the sixth aortic arterial arches, giving rise to the **pulmonary arteries**. A venous plexus surrounds the bronchial tree and drains into the left atrium

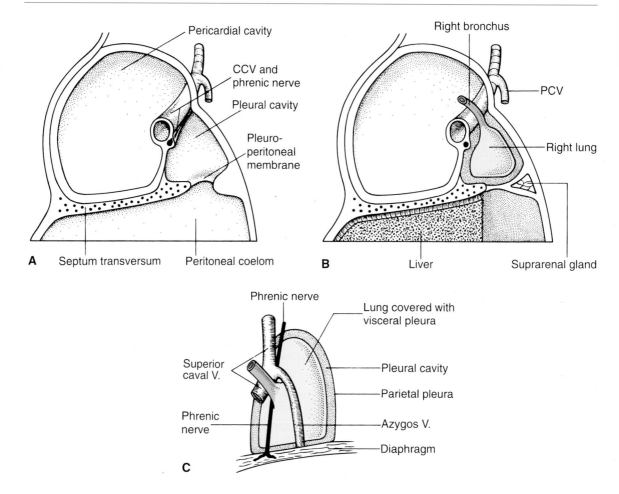

Figure 18.3. (A) Coelomic cavities of the right side at 7 weeks, with viscera removed. CCV, common cardinal vein forming pleuropericardial fold. (B) Same, with some viscera in place. PCV, right posterior cardinal vein (future azygos vein). (C) Anatomy at 12 weeks.

by way of **pulmonary veins**. The **bronchial arteries** originate as direct branches from the dorsal aortas.

Histogenesis of the Lungs

Bifurcation of the trachea produces two **primary bronchi**. The right primary bronchus divides into three **secondary** or **lobar bronchi**, which break up further within the three **lobes** of the right lung. The left one divides into two lobar bronchi to serve the two lobes of the left lung. The lobar bronchi divide in turn into **segmental bronchi** whose branches ultimately form the **bronchopulmonary segments** of the lungs.

During the middle trimester (middle 3 months of pregnancy), the lungs bear a histological resemblance to exocrine glands (*Figure 18.6*). They consist of bronchial subdivisions lined by cubical epithelium. During the 7th month, **respiratory bronchioles** become abundant, and progressively more of these terminate in **alveolar ducts** and **alveolar sacs**. The sacs are lined at first

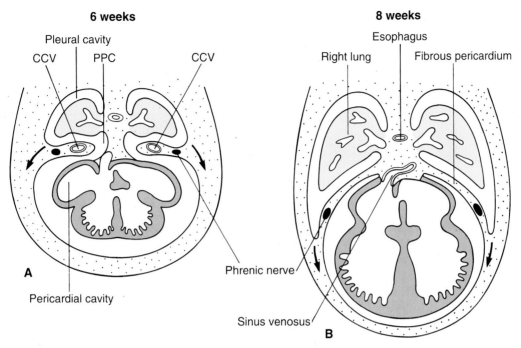

Figure 18.4. Transverse sections of thorax. (A) At 6 weeks. The phrenic nerves and common cardinal veins (CCV) occupy the pleuropericardial folds. PPC, pleuropericardial connection. (B) At 8 weeks. The phrenic nerves are embedded in the fibrous pericardium. Arrows in (A) and (B) indicate extension of pleural cavities.

by flattened, type 1 alveolar cells, destined to serve in gaseous exchange at the **blood–air barrier**. At the end of the 6th month, type 2 alveolar cells are also in evidence. The type 2 secrete **surfactant**, a detergent substance that lowers the surface tension at the interface between the alveolar epithelium and inspired air when the infant is born. When sufficient surfactant has been secreted into the alveolar sacs, the fetus becomes viable.

A significant threat to prematurely born infants – especially if born before the end of the 34th week – is *respiratory distress syndrome*. Because the production of surfactant is still insufficient, the fluid in the alveoli exerts so much tension that they cannot expand fully during inspiration and they tend to collapse during expiration.

Budding of fresh bronchioles, alveolar ducts, and alveolar sacs continues until the 8th or 9th year of postnatal life.

ESOPHAGUS

The esophagus extends from the lower limit of the pharynx to the stomach (*Figure 18.2E*). It is suspended from the posterior body wall by a *mesoesophagus* during the embryonic period. The short mesoesophagus of the midthoracic region can be identified in *Figure 18.4*. The lower end of the esophagus moves away from the vertebral column, yielding a longer dorsal mesentery (*Figure 18.7*, p.117).

The esophagus lengthens in company with the thoracic cavity as a whole. Pharyngeal arch mesoderm contributes striated muscle to its upper part, to be supplied by the recurrent laryngeal branches of the vagus nerves. Splanchnic mesoderm contributes smooth muscle to its lower part; this muscle is supplied by autonomic neurons derived from the neural crest.

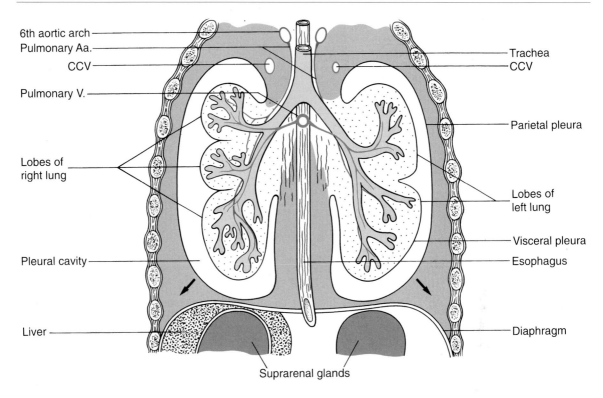

6th aortic arch
Pulmonary Aa.
CCV
Pulmonary V.

Trachea
CCV

Parietal pleura

Lobes of
right lung

Lobes of
left lung

Visceral pleura

Pleural cavity

Esophagus

Liver

Diaphragm

Suprarenal glands

Figure 18.5. Coronal section of the posterior mediastinum at 7 weeks. CCV, common cardinal vein. Arrows indicate directions of expansion of pleural cavities and lungs. The septum transversum has been incorporated into the diaphragm.

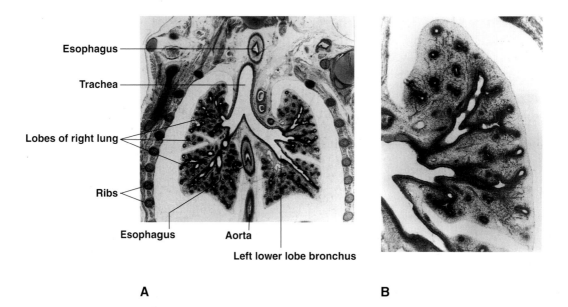

Esophagus

Trachea

Lobes of right lung

Ribs

Esophagus   Aorta

Left lower lobe bronchus

A   B

Figure 18.6. (A) Frontal section of thorax at 10 weeks. (B) Upper lobe of the left lung. (Carnegie Collection.)

DIAPHRAGM

Five elements contribute to the formation of the diaphragm, as follows (*Figure 18.7*):

• Prior to its descent along with the heart, the septum transversum lies opposite the third to fifth cervical somites. These somites are generally considered to contribute cells which later differentiate to form the musculature of the diaphragm. Such an arrangement accounts for the motor innervation of the diaphragm by

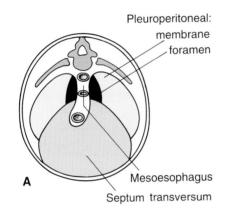

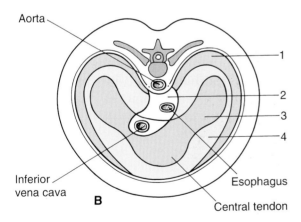

Figure 18.7. Diaphragm, viewed from above. (A) Embryonic. (B) Definitive. Component elements: 1, body wall; 2, mesoesophagus; 3, septum transversum; 4, pleuroperitoneal membrane. *Note*: The muscle fibers are derived from cervical somites.

the ventral rami of the third, fourth, and fifth cervical spinal nerves, in the form of the phrenic nerve. The phrenic nerve also provides sensory fibers to the upper and lower surfaces of the dome of the diaphragm.

• As noted in the account of the lungs, ventral extension of the pleural sac peels a layer of somatic mesoderm from the body wall to create the fibrous pericardium. The sacs enlarge in the vertical dimension as well, peeling off a layer which contributes connective tissue to the diaphragm. This contribution accounts for the presence of sensory fibers from the lower six intercostal nerves around the periphery.

• The mesentery of the esophagus contributes connective tissue to the diaphragm around the esophagus and inferior caval vein.

• The septum transversum gives rise to the fibrous tissue of the central tendon.

• The pleuroperitoneal membranes contribute connective tissue to the musculature surrounding the central tendon.

MALFORMATIONS

Lungs

A common anomaly (0.5% of the population) is the so-called *azygos lobe*, created by expansion of the upper lobe of the right lung on both sides of the posterior cardinal (azygos) vein – not merely on its lateral side. The condition is harmless; it is often detected during routine radiological investigation of the thorax.

Isomerism signifies a matching number of lobes (either two or three) in the two lungs, in association with dextrocardia (Chapter 17).

Pulmonary hypoplasia is characterized by smaller-than normal lungs showing reduced alveolar development. It is caused by compression. Examples of compression include oligohydramnios (deficient production of amniotic fluid), and congenital diaphragmatic hernia (see below).

Esophagus

Esophageal atresia is a failure of development of the esophagus. Typically, the upper part ends blindly, and the lower part has an open connection (fistula) with the trachea. Esophageal atresia is suspected in cases of *hydramnios*, where the amount of amniotic fluid is abnormally large. (The linkage between atresia and hydramnios is explained in Chapter 31.) Infants with esophageal atresia are unable to pass saliva to the stomach, and it regurgitates through the mouth within hours after birth. Possible associated anomalies include Fallot's tetralogy (Chapter 17), and ano-rectal agenesis (Chapter 23).

Diaphragm

The pleuroperitoneal foramen is normally sealed off in the late 6th or early 7th week. In 1 in 2000 of the population, the foramen persists, providing a channel for displacement of abdominal viscera into the thorax. The channel is known as the *foramen of Bochdalek*; in most cases it is found on the left side, perhaps because the liver provides support for the developing diaphragm on the right. An affected child is born with a *congenital diaphragmatic hernia*. Coils of intestine, and sometimes the stomach and spleen as well, enter the pleural cavity, with consequent compression of the lung and displacement of the heart.

In *congenital short esophagus*, the stomach is constricted into an hour-glass shape by the diaphragm. The upper part of the stomach occupies the thorax and receives its arterial blood supply from branches of the descending thoracic aorta, rather than from the celiac artery.

Congenital eventration of the diaphragm is a rare condition in which there is complete failure of muscle fibers to develop in the diaphragm on one side. The affected dome is represented only by an aponeurotic (fibrous) sheet riding high in the thorax, having been displaced by the normal pressure of the abdominal viscera.

EMBRYOLOGICAL TERMS

Laryngotracheal groove. Laryngotracheal tube. Respiratory diverticulum. Lung buds. Pleuropericardial fold. Pleuroperitoneal membrane. Mesoesophagus. *Azygos lobe. Pulmonary isomerism. Pulmonary hypoplasia. Esophageal atresia. Hydramnios. Congenital diaphragmatic hernia. Congenital short esophagus. Congenital eventration of the diaphragm.*

19

Abdomen: the foregut and its mesenteries

INTRODUCTION

In the middle of the 4th week of development, the alimentary tract comprises the endodermal *foregut*, *midgut* and *hindgut*, as illustrated in *Figure 19.1A*. The hindgut includes the *cloaca*, from which the allantois extends into the umbilical cord. The cloaca is not a purely alimentary structure; in due course it will form the bladder and urethra as well as the rectum.

The *hepatic diverticulum (liver bud)* is seen on day 24 as an endodermal thickening directly caudal to the septum transversum (*Figure 19.1B*).

By the end of the 4th week, the **pharynx**,

25 days

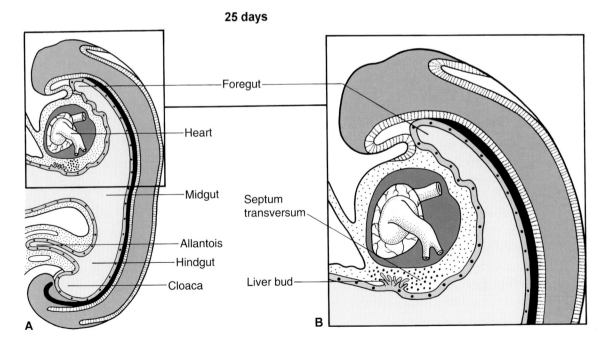

Figure 19.1. (A) Digestive system at 25 days. (B) Enlargement from (A).

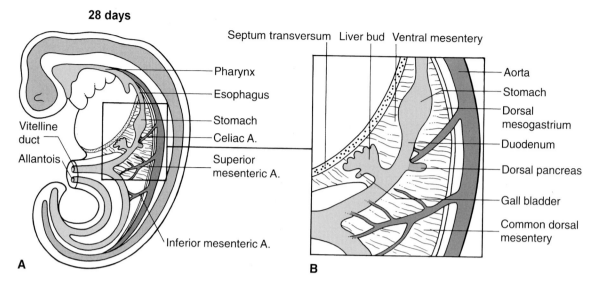

28 days

Figure 19.2. (A) Digestive system at 4 weeks. (B) Enlargement from (A).

esophagus and **stomach** can be identified (*Figure 19.2A*). The **definitive foregut** is defined henceforth as the segment of gut extending from the gastroesophageal junction to include the liver bud. It is supplied with blood by the **celiac artery**. The **superior mesenteric artery** supplies the midgut and the **inferior mesenteric artery** supplies the hindgut; the anatomical limits of midgut and hindgut are not yet defined.

LIVER AND GALL BLADDER

Immediately beyond the stomach is the **duodenum**, from which the liver bud grows into the ventral mesentery (*Figures 19.2B and 19.3*). The liver bud gives off the **gall bladder** before dividing into left and right hepatic buds. The stalk of the gall bladder bud becomes the **cystic duct**, and the stalks of the hepatic buds become the **hepatic ducts**. The **bile duct** is formed by the union of the conjoined hepatic ducts with the cystic duct (*Figure 19.4*).

The hepatic buds produce an anastomosing network of **hepatocytes**. The vitelline

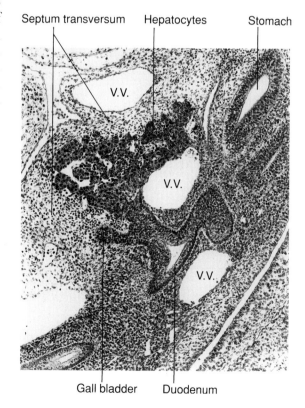

Figure 19.3. Hepatic bud at 25 days. VV, vitelline veins. (Carnegie Collection.)

veins spill into the interstices, forming the liver **sinusoids**. The ventral mesenchyme gives rise to the connective tissue of the liver, also to the **Kupffer cells** lining the sinusoids. Bile is secreted by the hepatocytes from the 13th week onward, and the contents of the intestine (known as *meconium*) acquire a dark green color.

The left hepatic bud forms the left lobe of the liver, also the caudate and quadrate lobes which belong, descriptively, to the right lobe of adult anatomy. The right hepatic bud forms the remainder of the right lobe.

The liver participates in hemopoiesis, in blood islands seeded there from the wall of the yolk sac. Hemopoiesis is especially active during the middle trimester of pregnancy. It normally ceases at full term, but it may resume in postnatal life in certain pathologic states (e.g. leukemia).

PANCREAS (Figure 19.4)

The pancreas has a dual origin from alimentary endoderm. A *ventral pancreas* arises from the stem of the hepatic diverticulum (future bile duct). A larger, *dorsal pancreas* arises from the duodenum and burrows into the dorsal mesogastrium.

Unequal growth of the dudodenal wall carries the bile duct, and with it the ventral pancreas, first to its dorsal and later to its left aspect. The ventral pancreas forms the **uncinate process** of the pancreas; the dorsal pancreas forms the **head**, **body** and **tail**.

The **main pancreatic duct** enters the duodenum in common with the bile duct. It is formed by take-over of the duct of the ventral pancreas by the duct of the dorsal pancreas. The stem of the original dorsal duct persists as the small **accessory pancreatic duct**.

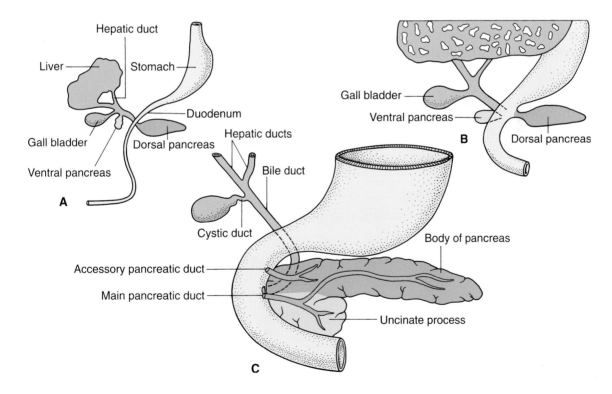

Figure 19.4. Development of duct systems of liver, gall bladder, and pancreas.

The intense mitotic activity of the duodenal epithelium in producing the hepatic and dorsal pancreatic diverticula, interrupts its lumen during the 5th and 6th weeks. By the end of the 7th week the definitive lumen is established by coalescence of intercellular spaces created by localized cellular death.

PORTAL VEIN

The portal system of veins drains the entire alimentary tract below the diaphragm. The portal vein proper develops from segments of the two vitelline veins, which fuse below, within and above the C-shaped duodenum (*Figure 19.5A*). As the third (horizontal) part of the duodenum becomes fixed to the posterior abdominal wall, the dorsal venous loop is lost at this level. At the level of the first part, the ventral loop is lost (*Figure 19.5B*). The splenic vein receives the inferior mesenteric vein and joins the middle anastomosis. Cranially, the vitelline veins form the left and right branches of the portal vein within the liver.

Ductus Venosus

During the 4th week, plates of cells growing from the liver bud tap the vitelline veins, thereby establishing the liver sinusoids. During the 5th week, the right umbilical vein shrinks and disappears while the left one enlarges to accommodate the entire return of blood from the placenta (*Figure 19.6A, B*).

During the 6th–8th weeks, a large vascular shunt diverts the oxygenated blood from the left umbilical to the right hepatic vein. This vascular shunt is the *ductus venosus (venous duct)* (*Figures 19.6C, 19.7 and 19.8*). The right vitelline vein also becomes linked to a *subcardinal vein* draining the kidneys, whereupon this segment of the right vitelline is known as the *hepatic portion of the inferior vena cava*. The upper part of the left vitelline vein disappears.

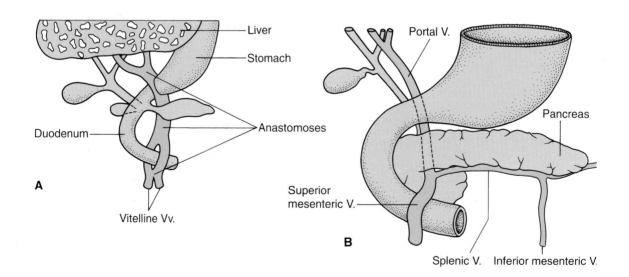

Figure 19.5. Transformation of the vitelline veins below the level of the liver.

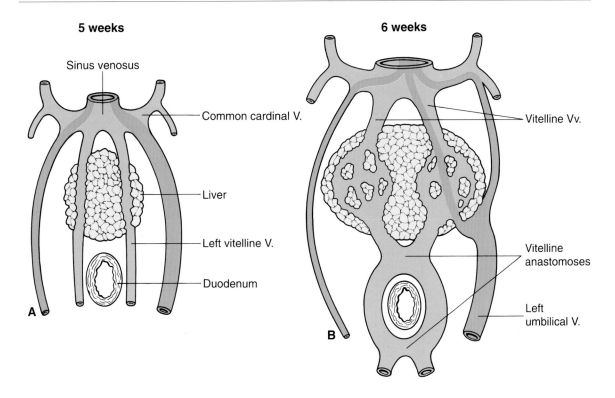

5 weeks

- Sinus venosus
- Common cardinal V.
- Liver
- Left vitelline V.
- Duodenum

A

6 weeks

- Vitelline Vv.
- Vitelline anastomoses
- Left umbilical V.

B

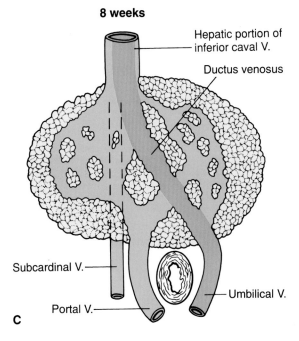

8 weeks

- Hepatic portion of inferior caval V.
- Ductus venosus
- Subcardinal V.
- Portal V.
- Umbilical V.

C

Figure 19.6. Scheme to show transformation of the vitelline and umbilical veins.

VENTRAL MESENTERY

The expanding liver divides the ventral mesentery into the **lesser omentum**, extending from liver to foregut, and the **falciform ligament**, extending from liver to anterior abdominal wall (*Figure 19.9*). Cephalic extension of the liver brings it into contact with the horizontal part of the septum transversum, which is the forerunner of the central tendon of the diaphragm. The **bare area** of the liver is created by direct contact with the septum transversum and with the right kidney and suprarenal gland. The right leaf of the falciform ligament forms the blunt **right triangular ligament**, and the left leaf forms the sharp **left triangular ligament**.

STOMACH AND OMENTAL BURSA

Initially, the ventral border of the stomach is attached to the ventral abdominal wall by

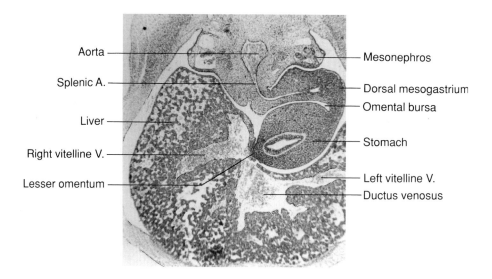

Figure 19.7. Transverse section at stomach level, early in the 6th week. (Carnegie Collection.)

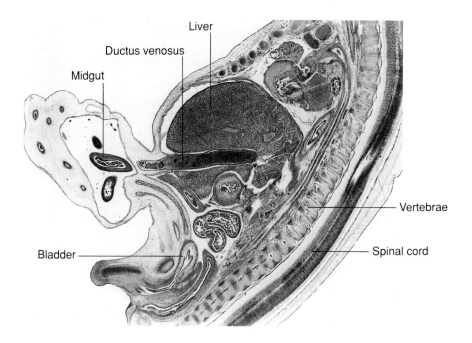

Figure 19.8. Median section of trunk at 10 weeks, showing the ductus venosus passing through the liver.

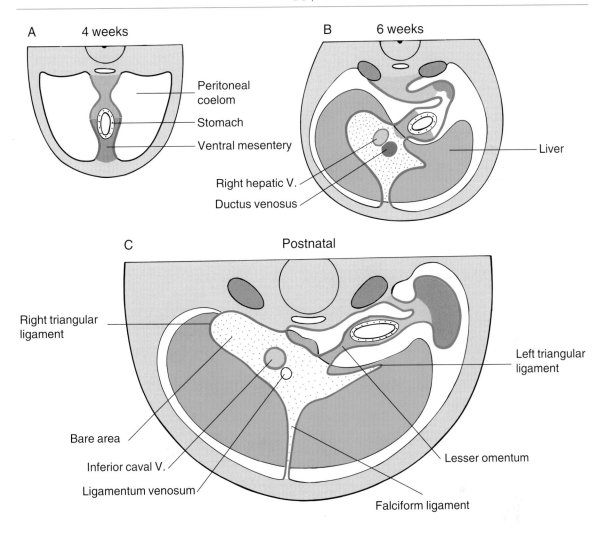

Figure 19.9. Transverse sections of the upper abdomen, showing transformation of the ventral mesentery.

the ventral mesentery, and the dorsal border is attached to the dorsal wall by the dorsal mesentery (*Figure 19.10A*). During the 5th and 6th weeks, the dorsal border elongates to form the convex **greater curvature**, the shorter ventral border persisting as the concave **lesser curvature**. At this time the stomach appears to undergo rotation through 90°, the lesser curvature being directed to the right and the greater curvature to the left (*Figure 19.10B*). A peritoneal pocket, the **omental bursa** (lesser sac of peritoneum), extends behind the stomach and into the dorsal mesogastrium, which is folded upon itself. The remainder of the peritoneal coelom is then known as the **greater sac**.

The positional changes of the curvatures of the stomach have two major effects. The liver, growing within the ventral mesentery, becomes a mainly right-sided organ; and the spleen, which develops within the dorsal mesentery, comes to lie on the left side.

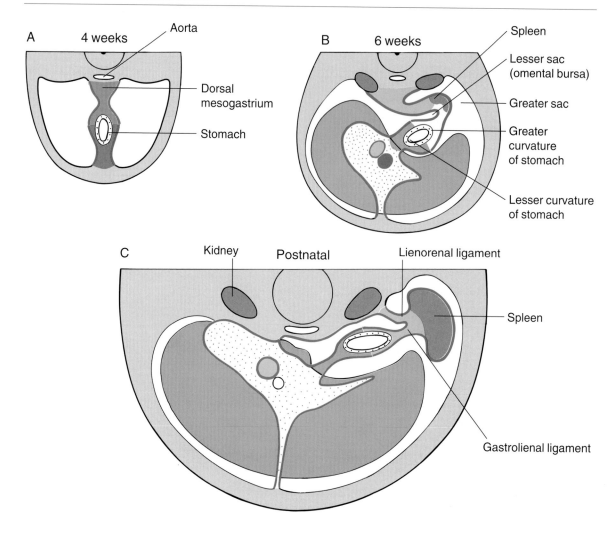

Figure 19.10. Transverse sections of upper abdomen, to show transformation of the dorsal mesogastrium.

SPLEEN

The primordium of the **spleen** makes its appearance during the 5th week as a focus of mesenchymal proliferation within the dorsal mesogastrium (*Figure 19.10B*). As it enlarges, it projects into the greater sac of peritoneum on the left side. The enlarging left kidney obliterates the overlying part of the greater sac. The left part of the dorsal mesogastrium then comprises the **gastrolienal ligament**, passing from stomach to spleen, and the **lienorenal ligament**, passing from spleen to left kidney (*Figure 19.10C*). The hilum of the spleen marks the left boundary of the omental bursa.

The spleen is seeded by hemopoietic cells from the wall of the yolk sac. It manufactures both red and white cells during the middle trimester of pregnancy.

The caudal part of the dorsal mesogastrium hangs down in front of the transverse colon. It becomes the greater omentum (see next chapter).

MALFORMATIONS

Biliary Tract

Anomalies of the cystic and hepatic ducts are commonplace and spring from the variable manner of branching of the original hepatic diverticulum. Rarely, the cystic branch of the diverticulum may fail altogether, with consequent *absence of the gall bladder*. The hepatic diverticulum or its branches may fail to acquire a lumen, leading to atresia of the biliary or cystic ducts. Biliary atresia leads to distension of the gall bladder and hepatic ducts, to pallor of the meconium, and to a progressively deepening jaundice after birth.

Duodenum

Failure of the duodenal lumen to become recanalized – *duodenal stenosis* – is a well-known cause of intestinal obstruction in the newborn. The obstruction occurs just beyond the opening of the bile duct. It is marked by persistent vomiting of bile-stained fluid within hours after birth.

Pancreas

Annular pancreas is a condition where the second part of the duodenum is surrounded by a ring of pancreatic tissue which may cause some degree of obstruction. A possible explanation is migration of the ventral pancreas around both sides of the duodenum, instead of merely migrating behind it.

EMBRYOLOGICAL TERMS

Hepatic diverticulum (liver bud). Ventral and dorsal pancreas. Ductus venosus. *Atresia of biliary or cystic ducts. Duodenal stenosis. Annular pancreas.*

20

Abdomen: midgut and common dorsal mesentery

At the time of appearance of the omental bursa, the vitelline duct is undergoing a rapid reduction in size. The attachment of the vitelline duct to the gut keeps the middle part of the intestinal tract close to the umbilicus (see *Figure 19.2*). The resultant U-shaped segment of intestine is the midgut loop.

The *division of the cloaca* must be mentioned at this point. In the 5 week embryo, the cloaca is the most caudal part of the hindgut, caudal to the opening of the allantois (*Figure 20.1A*). Cloacal endoderm is fused with surface ectoderm at the cloacal membrane. During the following 10 days, a mesodermal partition, the *urorectal septum*, divides the cloaca into *rectum* and *urogenital sinus* (*Figure 20.1B*).

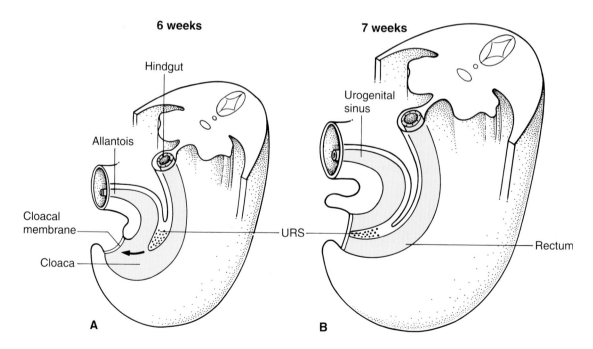

Figure 20.1. Division of the cloaca.

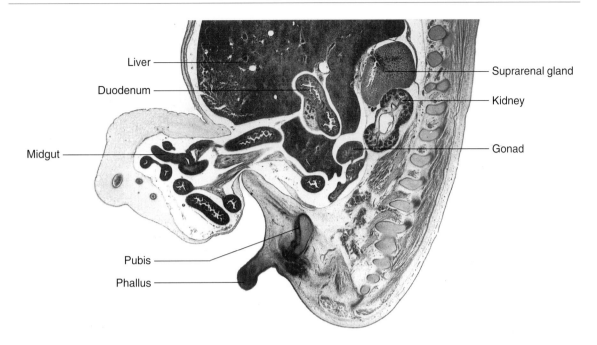

Figure 20.2. Median section of abdomen at 9 weeks, showing the physiological hernia of the midgut. (Carnegie Collection.)

MIDGUT

During the 6th week, the midgut lengthens to the extent that it can no longer be accommodated within the abdominal cavity. Room is found instead within the umbilical cord, producing the remarkable *physiological hernia of the midgut* (*Figure 20.2*).

Rotation of the Midgut

Even as it enters the umbilical cord, the midgut begins to twist on itself. The axis of rotation is provided by the superior mesenteric artery, which runs to the apex of the loop, beyond a swelling created by the developing **cecum** (*Figure 20.3*). When the viscera are observed from in front, the direction of rotation is counterclockwise. A rotation of 180° carries the caudal limb of the U to the left of the cranial limb and then above it. A further 90° of rotation carries the cecum and proximal **colon** to the right. At the same time, the original cranial limb is forming the **jejunum** and **ileum**.

By the 12th week, the capacity of the peritoneal coelom has increased substantially and the intestine slides back into the abdomen. The small intestine returns first and fills the central region. The colon comes next and forms a 'picture frame' around the periphery (*Figure 20.4A*). The cecum is the widest part of the gut and is held back until last. It enters the right side of the abdomen below the liver. Because the liver fills two-thirds of the abdominal cavity at this time, the cecum immediately takes up its proper position in the right iliac fossa. The colon passes obliquely across the abdomen as far as the spleen, an arrangement which holds good until the time of birth. Later, the liver undergoes a relative retreat and the oblique segment angulates where it crosses the duodenum (to which it has become fixed). The **ascending colon** then extends

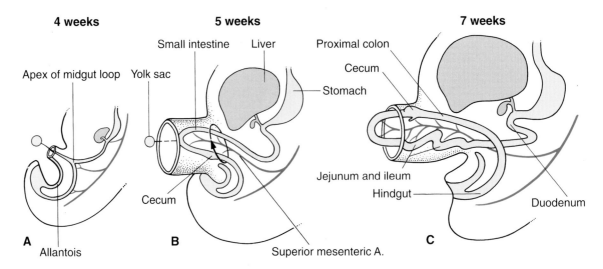

Figure 20.3. (A) Intestine at 4 weeks. (B) Entry of midgut loop into umbilical cord. Arrow indicates rotation of the midgut loop. (C) Rotation through 180° carries cecum and proximal colon to a cranial position.

from the cecum to the **hepatic flexure** at the point of angulation, and the **transverse colon** extends from there across to the **splenic flexure**. The **descending colon** and **sigmoid colon** pass down on the left side to reach the rectum.

trium becomes adherent to the transverse colon and mesocolon. The transverse mesocolon is then redefined to include this contribution, thereby placing the transverse colon and mesocolon in the posterior wall of the lesser sac.

FATE OF THE COMMON DORSAL MESENTERY

The attachment of the common dorsal mesentery to the posterior abdominal wall is greatly modified following return of the midgut loop into the abdominal cavity from the umbilical cord. The principal changes are shown in *Figures 20.4B* and *20.5*:

- The duodenum, ascending colon and descending colon become retroperitoneal. As a result, the common dorsal mesentery is divided into three parts, namely the **mesentery** (of the small intestine), **transverse mesocolon**, and the **sigmoid mesocolon**.
- The lower part of the dorsal mesogas-

THE APPENDIX (*Figure 20.6*)

The primitive cecum is conical. Its tip tapers into a narrow **vermiform appendix**. The cecum develops three teniae of longitudinal muscle continuous with those of the colon. The teniae converge on the appendix and invest it completely. A conical cecum with the appendix hanging from its tip is characteristic in the newborn; it is occasionally observed in adults (so-called *infantile appendix*). Normally, the right side of the cecum bulges progressively in postnatal life, the appendix being displaced to its left side. However, the three teniae continue to converge upon the root of the appendix – a point of interest to the surgeon when searching for it.

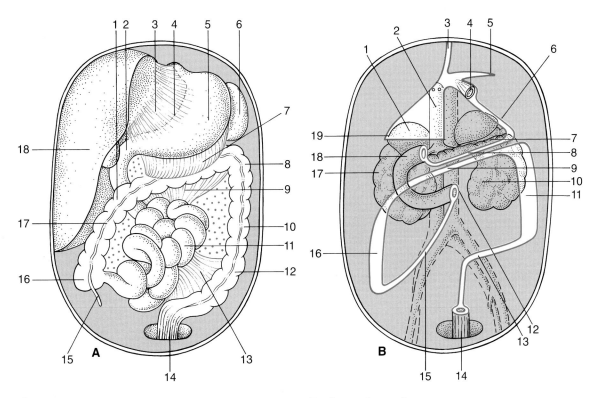

Viscera *in situ*

 1 Future hepatic flexure
 2 Duodenum
 3 Lesser omentum
 4 Lesser curvature of stomach
 5 Stomach
 6 Spleen
 7 Greater omentum
 8 Splenic flexure
 9 Transverse mesocolon
10 Desending colon
11 Small intestine
12 Sigmoid colon
13 Sigmoid mesocolon
14 Rectum
15 Appendix
16 Cecum
17 Ascending colon
18 Liver

Peritoneal attachments

 1 Suprarenal gland
 2 Inferior caval vein
 3 Falciform ligament
 4 Esophagus
 5 Left triangular ligament
 6 Lienorenal ligament
 7 Pancreas
 8 Greater omentum, fused with
 9 Transverse mesocolon
10 Kidney
11 Attachment of descending colon
12 Commencement of jejunum
13 Sigmoid mesocolon
14 Rectum
15 The mesentery
16 Attachment of ascending colon
17 Kidney
18 Duodenum
19 Right triangular ligament

Figure 20.4. Abdominal contents in late fetal life. (A) Viscera *in situ*. Blue dots indicate sites of fusion of mesenteries of duodenum, ascending and descending colon, with posterior abdominal wall. (B) Peritoneal attachments.

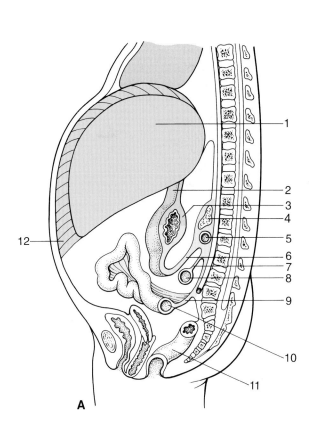

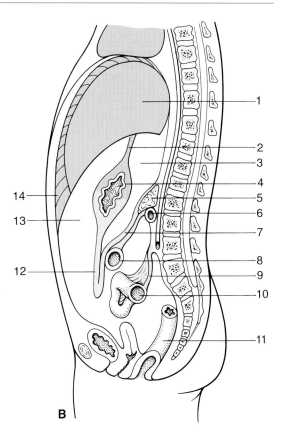

Fetal arrangement

1 Liver
2 Ventral mesogastrium
3 Stomach
4 Pancreas
5 Duodenum
6 Dorsal mesogastrium
7 Dorsal mesentery
8 Transverse colon
9 Dorsal mesentery
10 Sigmoid colon
11 Rectum
12 Ventral mesogastrium

Adult arrangement

1 Liver
2 Lesser omentum
3 Lesser sac

Figure 20.5. Sagittal sections of the abdomen. (A) Fetal. (B) Adult.

4 Stomach
5 Pancreas
6 Duodenum
7 Transverse mesocolon
8 Transverse colon
9 Sigmoid mesocolon
10 Sigmoid colon
11 Rectum
12 Greater omentum
13 Greater sac
14 Falciform ligament

MALFORMATIONS

Meckel's Diverticulum

In 2% of subjects a short, blind pocket projects from the ileum, about 60 cm from the ileocecal junction. This is *Meckel's diverticulum*, and it marks persistence of the proximal part of the vitelline duct. The epi-

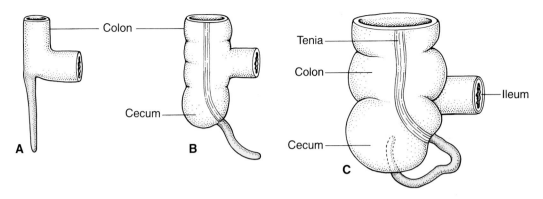

Figure 20.6. Vermiform appendix (blue). (A) At 10 weeks. (B) At birth. (C) Adult.

thelium of Meckel's diverticulum has the curious property of differentiating at times into gastric mucous membrane or pancreatic acini. Sometimes a remnant of the duct, or of a vitelline vessel, may persist in the form of a fibrous cord stretching from the ileum to the umbilicus. Coils of intestine may loop around such a cord and become obstructed at any time in postnatal life.

Subhepatic Appendix

Following reduction of the physiological hernia, the cecum and appendix are in intimate contact with the right lobe of the liver. Sometimes, during reduction of the relative size of the liver during fetal life, the cecum and appendix maintain this relationship and ascend to the upper abdomen. The end-result is a *subhepatic appendix*, which can present severe technical problems if it becomes inflamed. The condition does not (as some assert) represent 'failure of descent' of the cecum into the right iliac fossa.

Malrotation of the Midgut

Incomplete rotation of the midgut loop leaves the appendix in the center of the abdomen or even on the left side. *Reverse rotation* may be a sign of *situs inversus viscerum* ('inverted arrangement of the viscera'). Individuals with complete situs inversus have a mirror-image arrangement of the viscera, with the liver on the left side and the spleen on the right. They can easily be detected by the presence of *dextrocardia*, with an apex beat in the *right* fifth intercostal space.

Congenital Umbilical Hernia

Exomphalos is a condition where loops of intestine protrude through the umbilicus at birth. The hernial sac (wall) is formed by a loculus of peritoneum, covered externally by amnion.

EMBRYOLOGICAL TERMS

Rectum. Urogenital sinus. Midgut loop. Physiological hernia of the midgut. Rotation of the midgut. *Meckel's diverticulum. Subhepatic appendix. Exomphalos. Dextrocardia. Situs inversus viscerum.*

21

Abdomen: suprarenal glands, kidneys and inferior caval vein

DERIVATIVES OF THE INTERMEDIATE MESODERM

The intermediate mesoderm becomes detached from the paraxial and lateral plate mesoderm, and takes up a position on the posterior wall of the coelomic cavity beside the root of the dorsal mesentery (*Figure 21.1*).

The intermediate mesoderm gives rise to the following structures: the cortex of the suprarenal glands, the kidneys, the gonads and the genital ducts.

SUPRARENAL GLAND (*Figure 21.2*)

The suprarenal (adrenal) gland has a dual origin. The cortex develops from the intermediate mesoderm whereas the medulla is of ectodermal origin, from the neural crest.

Cortex

During the 5th postovulatory week, the suprarenal cortex makes an appearance at the level of the last two thoracic somites. The first collection of cells forms a thick, spherical, *fetal cortex*.

A second group of cells surrounds the first and forms the *definitive cortex*, which differentiates into the **zona glomerulosa** and **zona fasciculata**. The **zona reticularis** seems to originate from the outer part of the fetal cortex. The inner part of the fetal cortex persists throughout fetal life (accounting for the relatively large overall size of the fetal gland), but it degenerates shortly after birth.

Medulla

The **chromaffin cells** of the adrenal medulla are modified sympathetic ganglion cells. They are derived from cells of the neural crest which migrate into the interior of the gland from its medial aspect. They congregate in the center, around tributaries of the suprarenal vein, and receive direct synaptic contacts from preganglionic fibers emerging from the eleventh and twelfth thoracic segments of the spinal cord. The chief secretion of the chromaffin cells is epinephrine (adrenaline), which is liberated into the capillary bed surrounding the individual cells.

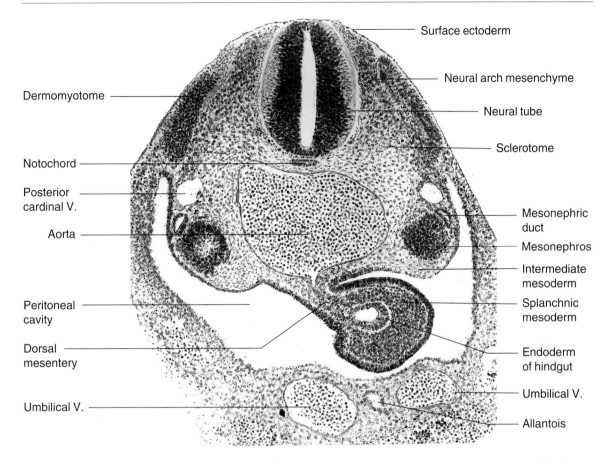

Figure 21.1. Transverse section through the caudal part of a 4-week embryo. (Carnegie Collection.)

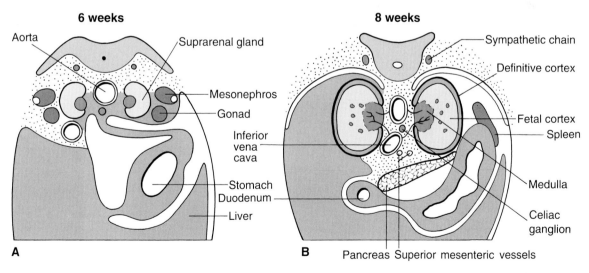

Figure 21.2. Transverse sections taken at the level of the suprarenal glands. Neural crest derivatives are shown in red.

KIDNEY

Three pairs of kidneys make an appearance in succession during development. All three originate in the intermediate mesoderm. The first kidney is the *pronephros*, which forms the permanent kidney of some fishes. The second is the *mesonephros*, which forms the permanent kidney of adult amphibia. The third is the *metanephros*, the permanent kidney of mammals.

Pronephros

In humans, the pronephros consists of nothing more than a few transient cell collections in the cervical region of the embryo early in the 4th week.

Mesonephros

The mesonephros is present during weeks 4–8. It consists of renal glomeruli fed by branches of the abdominal aorta, and renal tubules opening into the *mesonephric duct* (*Wolffian duct*) (*Figures 21.3* and *21.4*). The

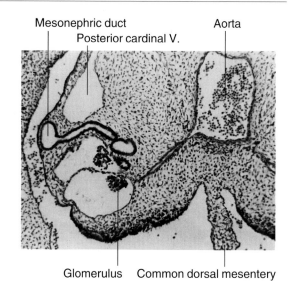

Figure 21.4. Mesonephros, early in the 6th week. (Carnegie Collection.)

Wolffian duct descends close to the surface of the intermediate mesoderm and opens into the cloaca.

As noted in Chapter 20, the cloaca becomes divided by a *urorectal septum* into *urogenital sinus* and **rectum** (*Figure 21.5A,B*). The urogenital sinus gives rise to the **bladder** and the **urethra** (*Figure 21.5C*). (Details of bladder and urethral development are in Chapter 23.)

Metanephros

The metanephros, or permanent kidney, develops from the intermediate mesoderm at sacral level. It is initially a pelvic organ. The collecting and secretory systems develop separately.

Collecting System

In the 5th week, a *ureteric bud* sprouts from the lower end of the Wolffian duct (*Figure 21.5A*). The bud burrows into the intermediate mesoderm behind the lower end of the

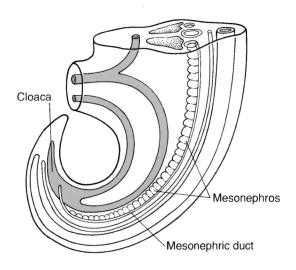

Figure 21.3. Mesonephros and mesonephric duct at 4 weeks.

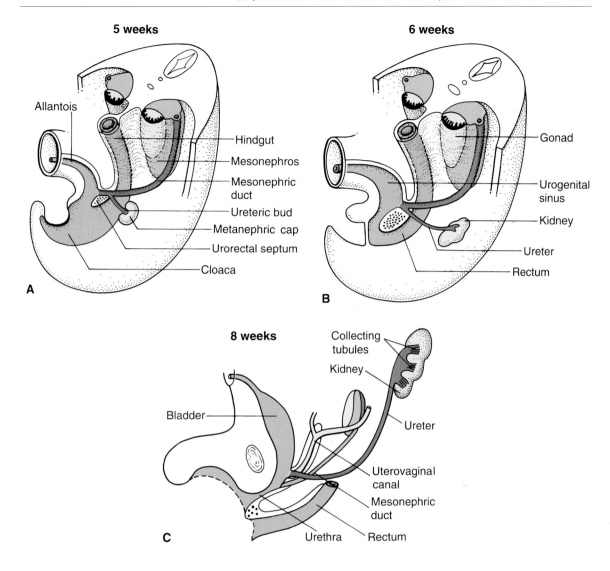

Figure 21.5. Early development of urinary system.

mesonephros. Its stalk acquires a lumen and becomes the **ureter** proper. The advancing bud hollows out to become the **renal pelvis**. The surrounding cells of the intermediate mesoderm multiply and invest the renal pelvis with a *metanephric cap* (*Figure 21.5A*).

The ureteric bud divides dichotomously to form successive generations of collecting tubules. The first four generations of tubules enlarge and coalesce to form the **major calyces** of the kidney. The second four generations coalesce to form the **minor calyces**. The minor calyces expand in cup-like fashion, each one receiving about 16 tubules of the ninth order. Tubules of the ninth to the sixteenth order persist as such to form the definitive **collecting tubules** of the kidney (*Figure 21.5C*).

The metanephric cap arranges itself in lobules around the minor calyces. Lobulation is still recognizable in the kidneys at birth.

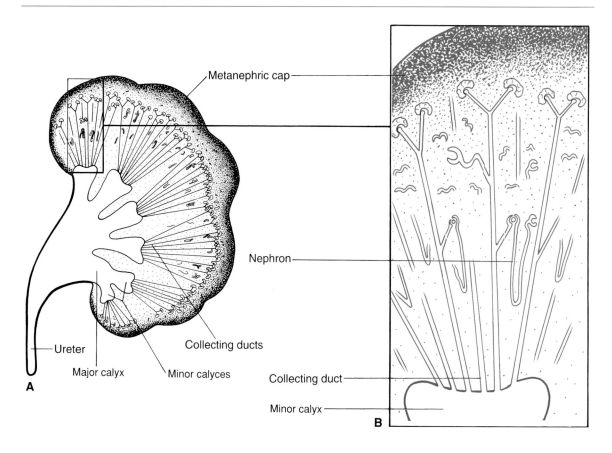

Figure 21.6. (A) Developing kidney at 12 weeks. (B) Enlargement from (A).

Secretory System

A cluster of metanephric cells forms at the tip of each collecting tubule (*Figure 21.6*). The cluster differentiates into a **nephron**, comprising Bowman's capsule, proximal convoluted tubule, loop of Henle, and distal convoluted tubule. Bowman's capsule is invaginated by a capillary tuft to complete the renal corpuscle. Each distal tubule opens into the *side* of the collecting tubule that induced the nephron. By this time the *tip* of the tubule has grown further into the in termediate mesoderm, to induce a succession of further nephrons in the same manner.

Ascent of the Kidneys

At first the kidneys lie in front of the sacrum, and the renal corpuscles are fed by branches of the internal iliac artery. Because of differential growth rates of skeletal and visceral elements in the pelvis and abdomen, the kidneys ascend from the pelvis during the 6th week (*Figures 21.7* and *21.8A*), and come into contact with the suprarenal glands by the 8th week (*Figure 21.8B*). By the 10th week the kidneys are in their final position, overlapping the last rib (*Figure 21.9*).

As they ascend, the kidneys are supplied successively from the common iliac arteries and the lower end of the aorta, and finally by the definitive renal arteries.

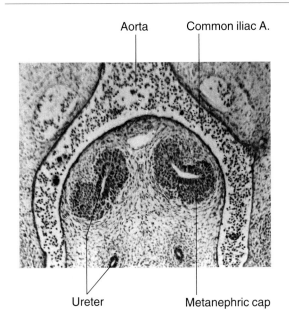

Aorta Common iliac A.

Ureter Metanephric cap

Figure 21.7. Metanephros pair ascending from the pelvis, at 6 weeks. (Cambridge Collection.)

Function of the Fetal Kidneys

The metanephros is functional from mid-gestation onwards. Urine is excreted into the amniotic cavity and much of it is transferred across the amnion to the placenta. Some is swallowed by the fetus, absorbed from the intestine, and its waste products taken to the placenta by the fetal circulation, for disposal into the maternal blood.

INFERIOR CAVAL VEIN

The development of the inferior caval vein (ICV) is complex. As many as five pairs of longitudinal channels develop on the posterior abdominal wall at different times.

The principal feature is the replacement of the posterior cardinal veins by two new channels – right subcardinal and right supracardinal (*Figure 21.10*). Paired *subcardinal veins* appear on the medial side of the two mesonephroi and anastomose freely with

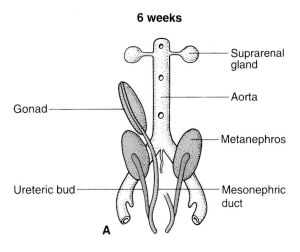

6 weeks

Suprarenal gland

Gonad

Aorta

Metanephros

Ureteric bud

Mesonephric duct

A

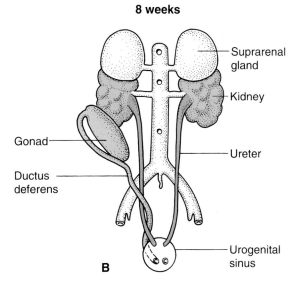

8 weeks

Suprarenal gland

Kidney

Gonad

Ureter

Ductus deferens

Urogenital sinus

B

Figure 21.8. Renal ascent. (A) At 6 weeks. (B) At 8 weeks.

the posterior cardinals. The right subcardinal sends a vascular bud, called the *hepatic segment* (of the ICV) to join the hepatocardiac channel. The subcardinal veins anastomose in front of the abdominal aorta. Paired *supracardinal veins* develop in the interval between the posterior cardinals and the subcardinals, and they are linked to both. The renal and gonadal veins enter the supracardinal veins.

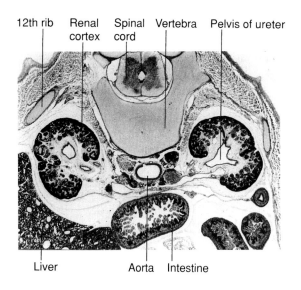

Figure 21.9. Kidneys in their final position, at 10 weeks. (Cambridge Collection.)

MALFORMATIONS

Kidney

Solitary kidney (unilateral renal agenesis) is sufficiently common (0.1% of the population) to require exclusion whenever surgical removal of a diseased kidney is contemplated. The cause may lie in failure of development of the ureteric bud or of the Wolffian duct from which the bud normally arises. In the latter case the ductus deferens (in a male) is absent on the affected side, and the testis is sometimes absent as well.

Bilateral renal agenesis (absence of both kidneys) occurs in 1 in 6000 live births. It is always suspected when the amount of amniotic fluid is very small (*oligohydramnios*). Fetal electrolytic stability is not impaired, being

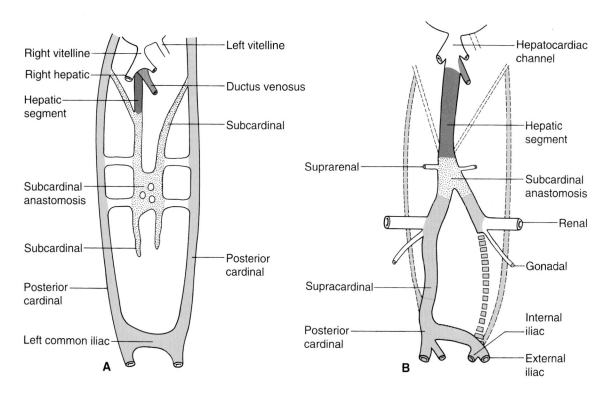

Figure 21.10. Diagrams showing development of the inferior caval vein. Five segments are depicted in (B).

controlled by placental exchange. The surface of the fetus is molded by pressure from the uterus (in the absence of amniotic fluid), producing a flattened face, low-set ears and deformity of the feet (Potter syndrome). Infants thus afflicted will survive for only a few days after birth unless peritoneal dialysis is undertaken. Pulmonary hypoplasia (from uterine compression of the thorax) is an added threat to life.

Polycystic kidney disease takes several different forms, with different pathologies and patterns of inheritance. The two main forms are known clinically as *infantile* and *adult*. The former is identified in infancy, being manifested by grossly enlarged, spongy kidneys, together with cystic changes in the liver and pancreas. The latter, although congenital, is usually detected in young adults presenting with symptoms of renal failure, or with hypertension of renal origin.

Ectopia of one or both kidneys is a consequence of failure of ascent to a normal level. An extreme form is that of a *pelvic kidney*, where one kidney remains beside the bladder and is fed by the internal iliac artery.

Horseshoe kidneys are produced by fusion of the lower poles prior to emergence of the embryonic kidneys from the pelvis. Ascent of the fused kidneys is arrested by the inferior mesenteric artery.

An *aberrant renal artery* commonly supplies the lower pole separately, from the aorta. The renal artery normally supplies five end arteries to the kidney, one to each of five tissue segments. An aberrant artery will supply one of the segments.

EMBRYOLOGICAL TERMS

Fetal suprarenal cortex. Pronephros. Mesonephros. Mesonephric duct. Metanephros. Ureteric bud. Metanephric cap. Renal ascent. Subcardinal veins. Supracardinal veins. *Bilateral renal agenesis. Polycystic kidney disease. Ectopic kidney. Pelvic kidney. Horseshoe kidneys. Aberrant renal artery.*

22

Pelvis and perineum: reproductive systems

EARLY GONADAL DEVELOPMENT

The gonad can be identified around the end of the 5th week, in the form of a thickening on the medial aspect of the ridge formed by the mesonephros (*Figure 22.1*). This new *gonadal ridge* is formed by thickening of the coelomic epithelium, and of the underlying intermediate mesoderm. The gonadal ridge and mesonephros together constitute the *urogenital ridge*.

The principal (or only) function of the thickened surface epithelium seems to be to liberate a chemical substance that attracts *primordial germ cells*. About 100 can be identified during the 4th week, on the surface of the caudal part of the yolk sac (*Figure 22.1A*). One or more may be already segregated within the morula, reaching the wall of the yolk sac during gastrulation. At any rate it is clear that one of the first duties of the embryoblast is to set aside the cell line that will contribute to the next human generation.

As soon as the gonad appears, the primordial germ cells migrate into the interior of the urogenital ridge (*Figures. 22.1B* and *22.2*). During the 6th and 7th weeks, they are enclosed by columns of epithelial cells derived from mesonephric tubules. The cell columns are known as *sex cords* (*Figure 22.3*).

Up to the end of the 7th week, the histological appearances are the same in male and female embryos, and the gonads are described as '*indifferent*'. Sexual differentiation (*sexual dimorphism*) of the gonads begins during the 8th week (see later).

'INDIFFERENT' GENITAL DUCTS

At the end of the 'indifferent' period, the embryo possesses two pairs of genital ducts (*Figure 22.3*). The mesonephric ducts are forerunners of the male ducts, and the paramesonephric ducts are forerunners of the female ones. Each *paramesonephric (Müllerian) duct* commences as a funnel-shaped invagination of the coelomic epithelium at the cephalic end of the mesonephros. The blind end of the duct burrows in a caudal direction, becoming canalized from above as it does so. At the lower end of the mesonephros the duct passes medially, ventral to the mesonephric duct, and descends in contact with its opposite number. The

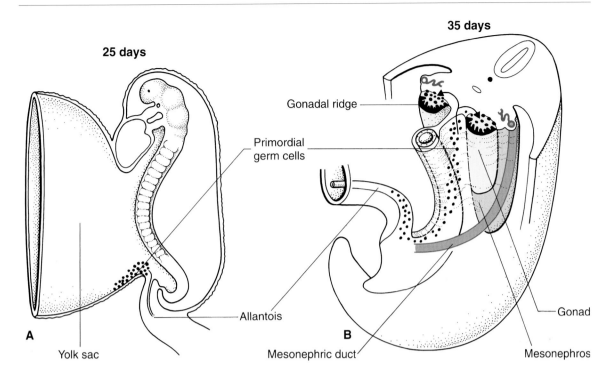

Figure 22.1. Migration of primordial germ cells during the 4th and 5th weeks. Arrows in (B) denote entry into gonads.

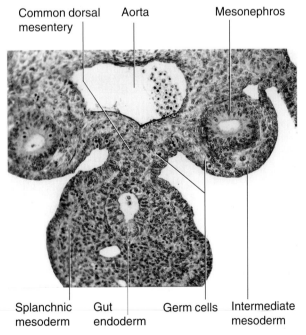

Figure 22.2. Transverse section of an early 5th-week embryo, showing germ cells traveling to the urogenital ridge. (Carnegie Collection, courtesy of Dr E. Witschi.)

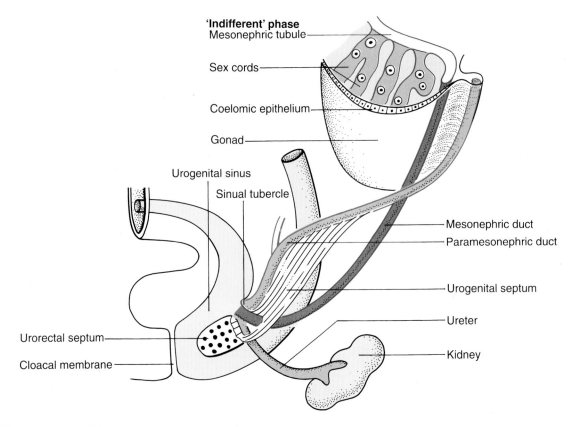

Figure 22.3. Indifferent gonad and genital ducts at 4 weeks.

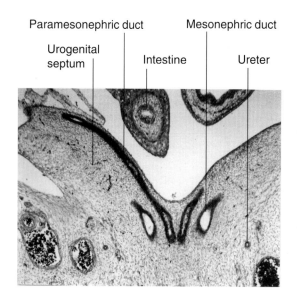

Figure 22.4. Frontal section of lower abdomen at 7 weeks. (Cambridge Collection.)

paired paramesonephric ducts terminate by abutting against the dorsal wall of the urogenital sinus, where they form a *sinual tubercle* (*Figure 22.3*).

Each Müllerian duct becomes suspended from the urogenital ridge by a short mesentery, and union of the two mesenteries creates a complete transverse partition, the *urogenital septum*, between the urogenital sinus and the rectum (*Figures 22.3, 22.4*).

SEXUAL DIMORPHISM

In male embryos, the short arm of the Y chromosome contains a gene responsible for production of a *testis-determining factor* (TDF). In the presence of TDF, the gonad will become a testis; otherwise the gonad will become an ovary.

Testis and Male Genital Duct

Around day 50, the intermediate mesoderm forms a fibrocellular shell, the **tunica albuginea**, beneath the surface epithelium (*Figure 22.5A*). The sex cords become *testicular cords*, and the primordial germ cells become *prospermatogonia* (*Figure 22.6A*). (Prospermatogonia remain dormant until puberty, when they become mature **spermatogonia** prior to commencing mitotic activity.) The testicular cords are segregated into lobules by **testicular septa** extending into the interior from the tunica albuginea. The inner ends of the cords are linked together in a network, the **rete testis** (*Figure 22.7*).

Two sets of endocrine cells are seen within the lobules:

- **Sustentacular cells** (*Sertoli cells*) are the most numerous cell type in the testicular

cords at this time (*Figure 22.6A*). The earliest function of Sertoli cells is to liberate a *Müllerian duct inhibitory factor* into the fetal circulation. The effect of this hormone is a regression of the paramesonephric ducts during the 9th week. The only constant representative of the paramesonephric ducts in later life in males is the **prostatic utricle** (*utriculus masculinus*) (*Figure 22.8B*).
- **Interstitial cells** (*Leydig cells*) arise from the mesenchymal stroma within the testicular lobules (*Figure 22.6A*). Leydig cells secrete *testosterone* into the fetal circulation. This hormone causes 6–12 mesonephric tubules, and the mesonephric duct, to survive and grow. The tubules form the **efferent ductules** connecting the rete testis to the head of the epididymis (*Figure 22.7*). The Wolffian duct itself forms the **duct of the epididymis**, the **ductus (vas) deferens**, the **seminal vesicle**, and the **ejaculatory duct** (*Figure 22.8A,B*).

In *females*, the Wolffian duct degenerates by a process of programmed cell death, without

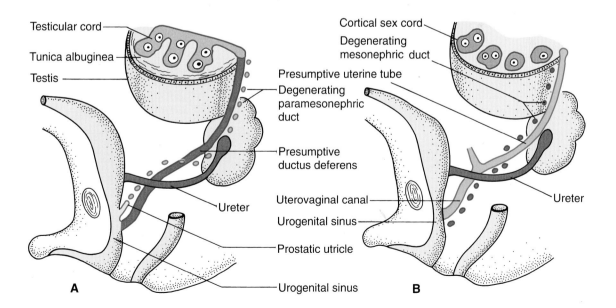

Figure 22.5. Early sexual differentiation. (A) Male. (B) Female.

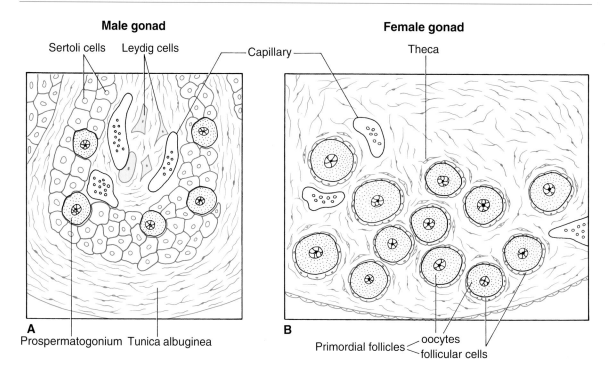

Figure 22.6. Microscopic appearance of the outer part of the gonads at 15 weeks.

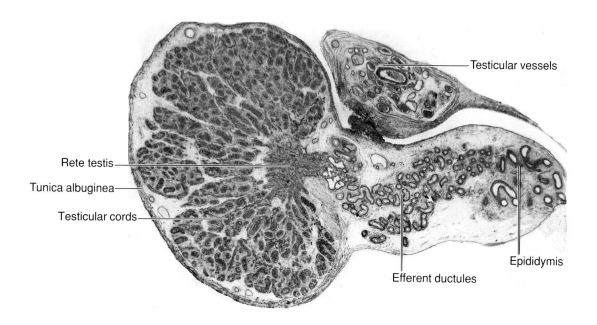

Figure 22.7. Transverse section of testis and related structures, at 20 weeks T. alb., tunica albuginea. (University of Washington Collection.)

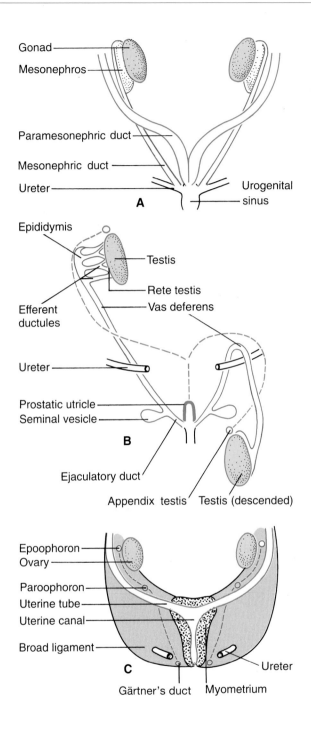

Figure 22.8. Diagrams showing fate of mesonephric and paramesonephric ducts. (A) Indifferent phase. (B) Male reproductive tract. Paramesonephric ducts are indicated by the dashed line. The appendix testis is a pin-head cyst commonly seen atop the testis in adults. (C) Female reproductive tract. Mesonephric remnants (red) include tubules/cysts near the ovary, and beside the cervix.

any hormonal influence from the ovary. Cystic or tubular remnants of the duct are normally found in the broad ligament in later life (*Figure 22.8C*) and are recognized as a source of *parovarian cysts*. Gynecologists refer to the mesonephric (Wolffian) duct as Gärtner's duct; hence their term *Gärtner's cyst* for a remnant sometimes found beside the cervix or vagina.

Ovary and Female Genital Duct

In the absence of a Y chromosome, the sex cords accumulate progressively in the outer region (cortex), and no tunica albuginea develops there (*Figure 22.6B*). The cortex becomes filled with **primordial follicles** comprising (a) **oocytes** derived from primordial germ cells, (b) an inner shell of **follicular cells** derived from cell-cord epithelium, and (c) an outer, connective tissue shell, the **theca**, derived from the intermediate mesoderm.

The number of primordial follicles reaches its maximum of 6–7 million around the 15th week. Through programmed cell death (*follicular atresia*), the number declines steeply later on. Two years after birth (*Figure 22.9*), about 1 million remain and, at puberty, about 0.3 million.

The paramesonephric ducts display upper vertical, intermediate oblique, and lower vertical segments (*Figure 22.8A*). In females, the upper and middle segments form the lining epithelium of the uterine tubes. The lower segments fuse with each other during the 9th or 10th week to form the *uterovaginal canal*, which in turn forms the lining epithelium of the **body** and **cervix** of the uterus (*Figures 22.10C* and *22.11*). The ducts also contribute to the vagina (see Chapter 23).

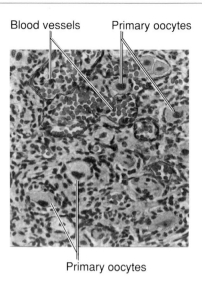

Blood vessels   Primary oocytes

Primary oocytes

Figure 22.9. Ovarian cortex of a 2-year-old girl. (University of Washington Collection, courtesy of Dr Charles Mottet.)

The muscular wall of the uterine tube, and of the uterus (**myometrium**) is added by the adjacent splanchnic mesoderm.

DESCENT OF THE GONADS

While sexual differentiation is commencing during the 8th week, a mesenchymal strand, known as the *gubernaculum* ('rudder') links the lower pole of the gonad to the lower end of the abdominal wall. The muscles of the abdominal wall are differentiating from the somatic mesoderm at this time (Chapter 11). The presence of gubernacular mesenchyme produces a *defect* in the musculature which is the forerunner of the **inguinal canal**.

Testicular Descent

During the 9th to 12th weeks, the testis descends a little, moving from the lumbar region into the iliac fossa (*Figure 22.10B*).

7 weeks

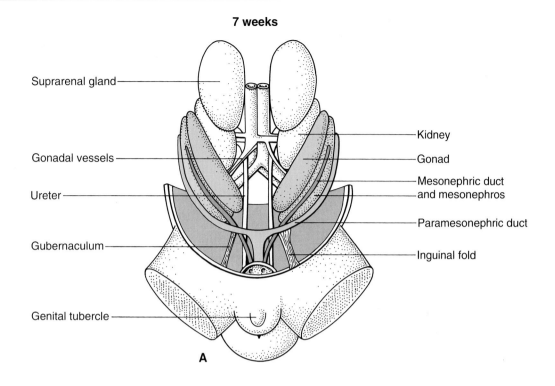

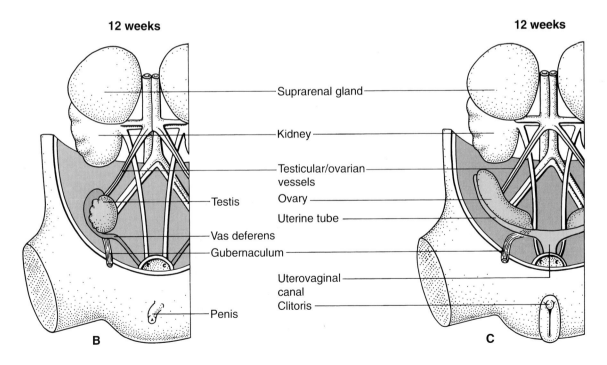

Figure 22.10. (A) Indifferent (bisexual) reproductive tract. (B) Male and (C) female reproductive tract at end of first trimester.

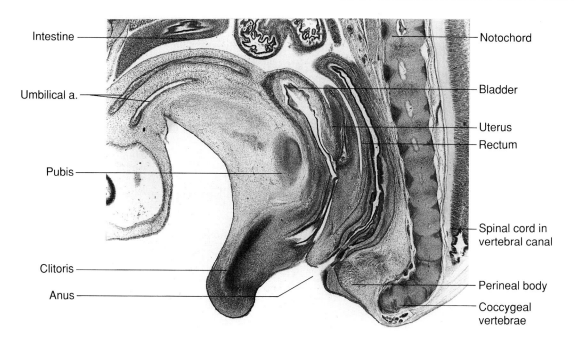

Figure 22.11. Median section of female pelvis at 9 weeks. (Carnegie Collection.)

This movement is usually attributed to growth of the vertebral column and pelvic bones, but an anchoring effect by the gubernaculum is also likely.

After the 18th week, the gubernaculum is swollen because of water uptake by its own intercellular matrix. It acquires the jelly-like consistency of an umbilical cord. During the 25th to 30th weeks it is as thick as the testis and epididymis combined, and it dilates the inguinal canal sufficiently to permit passage of the testis (with attached epididymis) before the end of the 30th week. A pocket of peritoneum, the *processus vaginalis*, hangs over the gubernaculum like an apron. The testis now lies in the subcutaneous tissue above the inguinal ligament.

During the next 5 weeks the gubernaculum shrinks and disappears. The processus vaginalis extends into the scrotum and the testis descends behind it. The final descent into the scrotum, is usually completed before birth but may take place during the first postnatal year. It is attributed to the activity of an as yet unidentified hormone. The ductus deferens and the testicular vessels, nerves and lymphatics accompany the testis; collectively, they constitute the **spermatic cord**.

The processus vaginalis is normally obliterated within the inguinal canal after the testis has passed through. Its blind lower extremity forms the **tunica vaginalis** covering the testis.

Ovarian Descent

The ovary is attached by a short mesentery (the **mesovarium**) to the back of the broad ligament of the uterus. It descends to the false pelvis by the 12th week (*Figure 22.10C*); later, it enters the true pelvis, being attached to the back of the broad ligament of the uterus. The gubernaculum of the ovary gains a secondary attachment to the upper corner of the uterus. Thus anchored, the gubernaculum elongates greatly, giving rise to the **round ligament of the uterus**. The segment passing from ovary to uterus forms the **ligament of the ovary**.

MALFORMATIONS

Testicular Descent

Abnormalities of testicular descent are of two kinds:

- In *incomplete descent*, the testes are arrested somewhere along the normal pathway. In *cryptorchism* (Greek, *kryptos*, 'hidden'), the testes remain within the abdomen. More commonly, they are 'canalicular' (in the inguinal canal) or 'high scrotal'. Incompletely descended testes are poorly developed.
- In *maldescent* (*ectopia*), a testis has taken up a position outside the normal pathway of descent. An ectopic testis may be found on the lower abdominal wall, in the perineum, or in the upper part of the thigh.

Persistence of the processus vaginalis takes three principal forms:

- Complete persistence provides a *congenital hernial sac* (*Figure 22.12A*) into which loops of intestine protrude during fetal life or infancy.
- The serous sac may be sealed off from the peritoneal cavity, but fluid accumulating within it produces a *hydrocele* around the testis (*Figure 22.12B*).
- The sac may be sealed off above and below, but distension with fluid in between forms a *hydrocele of the spermatic cord* (*Figure 22.12C*).

Female Genital Tract

A variety of malformations of the female genital tract may be encountered, based upon varying degrees of failure of union of the paramesonephric ducts:

- The least severe form is an *arcuate uterus*, which is flat-topped instead of having a convex fundus. Pregnancy in an arcuate uterus tends to result in an abnormal 'lie' of the fetus (for example, a transverse lie).
- More severe is a *bicornuate uterus*, where two uterine canals open into a common cervical canal.
- Most severe (and very rare) is a *septated uterus*, which is completely divided by a median septum; the vagina may be single or duplicated.

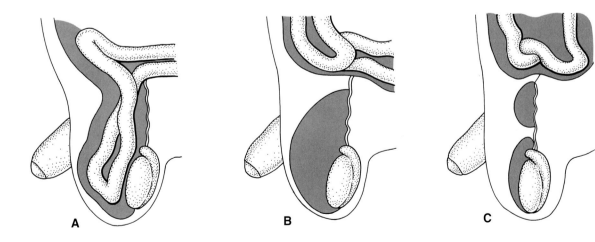

Figure 22.12. (A) Congenital hernial sac. (B) Hydrocele. (C) Hydrocele of the spermatic cord.

EMBRYOLOGICAL TERMS

Gonadal ridge. Urogenital ridge. Primordial germ cell. Sex cords. 'Indifferent' gonad. Sexual dimorphism. Paramesonephric duct. Sinual tubercle. Testicular cords. Prosper-matogonia. Oogonia. Primordial follicles. Follicular atresia. Gubernaculum. Processus vaginalis. *Arcuate uterus. Bicornuate uterus. Septated uterus. Incomplete descent of testis. Cryptorchism. Maldescent of testis (ectopia). Congenital hernial sac. Hydrocele. Hydrocele of the spermatic cord.*

23

Pelvis and perineum: vagina, bladder and urethra, external genitalia

BLADDER AND URETHRA

Figure 23.1 shows the visceral relationships in the caudal part of the trunk at 5 weeks. The caudal mesoderm, which was brought to the ventral aspect of the embryo during formation of the tail fold, fills the interval between the umbilicus and the cloacal membrane. Most of it remains here in the form of a midline swelling, the *genital tubercle*. Some of the caudal mesoderm migrates around the sides of the allantois and forms the *urorectal septum*, in a pocket between the allantois and the hindgut. The caudal end of the mesonephric duct is absorbed, giving the ureter a direct opening into the cloacal chamber.

During the 6th week (*Figure 23.1B*), the genital tubercle elongates as the *phallus*, forerunner of the penis in males and of the clitoris in females. The urorectal septum grows in the direction of the cloacal membrane. The mesonephric duct has begun to migrate caudally along the dorsal wall of the cloaca.

The anatomy at 8 weeks is shown in *Figure 23.2*. The urorectal septum fused with the cloacal membrane during the 7th week, creating the *urogenital sinus* and the *rectum*. The cloacal membrane was divided into a *urogenital membrane* and an *anal membrane*. The two membranes rupture at the end of the 7th or early in the 8th week. The mesoderm of the urorectal septum persists thereafter as the fibromuscular **perineal body**. The former site of attachment of the anal membrane lies in the floor of a shallow *anal pit*.

The urogenital sinus (UGS) is described as having three parts: a *vesical part*, above the level of entry of the mesonephric ducts, an intermediate, narrow, *pelvic part*, and a *phallic part* extending ventrally beneath the phallus.

The vesical part of the UGS expands to form the *primitive bladder*, which receives the two ureters. The **definitive bladder** is established by the differentiation of a coat of smooth muscle from the investing mesoderm.

Derivatives of the pelvic part of the UGS are included in *Figure 23.3*. In *males*, this part forms the lining epithelium of the **prostatic and membranous components of the urethra**. Small glandular outgrowths from the

5 weeks

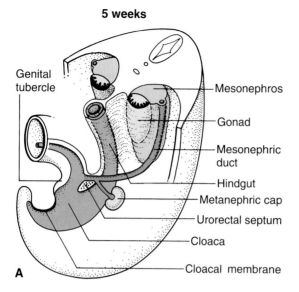

6 weeks

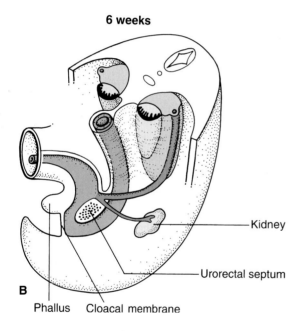

Figure 23.1. Early urogenital system.

8 weeks

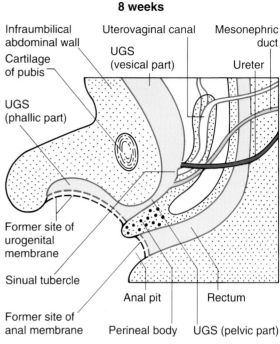

Figure 23.2. Sagittal section following complete division of the cloaca. UGS, urogenital sinus.

The phallic part of the UGS is considered together with the external genitalia, below.

VAGINA

At the point of contact between the mesoderm of the conjoint paramesonephric ducts and the endoderm of the urogenital sinus, mesodermal and endodermal cells together form a *sinual tubercle (Müllerian eminence)* (*Figure 23.2*). The tubercle gives rise to a *vaginal plate*, which lengthens by migrating in a caudal direction, along the dorsal wall of the urogenital sinus. The lumen of the vagina is formed by canalization of the vaginal plate from below upwards. The lumen extends around the cervix to establish the vaginal fornices. The **hymen** is a partition between the vagina proper and the vestibule.

prostatic urethra become surrounded by fibromuscular connective tissue developing from the splanchnic mesoderm, to complete the **prostate gland**. In *females*, the pelvic part forms the **epithelium of the entire urethra**, together with the **paraurethral glands**.

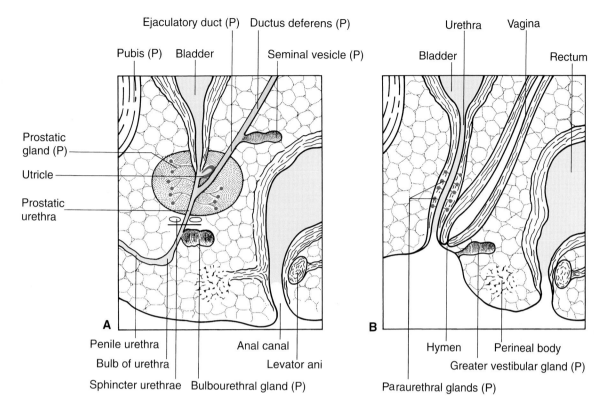

Figure 23.3. Sagittal sections of pelvic organs at about 20 weeks. (A) Male. (B) Female. Where structures are paired (P), the right (far side) members are represented. The sphincter urethrae muscle surrounds the membranous urethra.

Clinical and experimental evidence indicate that the upper two-thirds of the vaginal epithelium are derived initially from Müllerian (paramesonephric) mesoderm, and the lower one-third from sinus endoderm (*Figure 23.4B*). The vagina becomes lined throughout by stratified squamous epithelium.

folds derived from the adjacent mesenchyme. Lateral to these the mesenchyme forms paired *genital swellings* as well.

The fate of the urogenital folds and genital swellings is quite different in the two sexes. In males, under androgenic hormonal stimulation, the matching pairs come together in the midline. In females, they stay apart.

EXTERNAL GENITALIA

Indifferent Stage (Figure 23.5A)

Examination of the perineum early in the 3rd month shows no evidence of sexual divergence. The phallic urethra is an open *urethral groove*, flanked by paired *urogenital*

Male External Genitalia (Figure 23.5B,C)

Under testicular hormonal influence, the phallus in male fetuses elongates progressively to form the **penis**. The urogenital folds unite below the urethral groove to complete the **spongy urethra**. The line of union of the urogenital folds is marked by a **urethral raphe** in the midline.

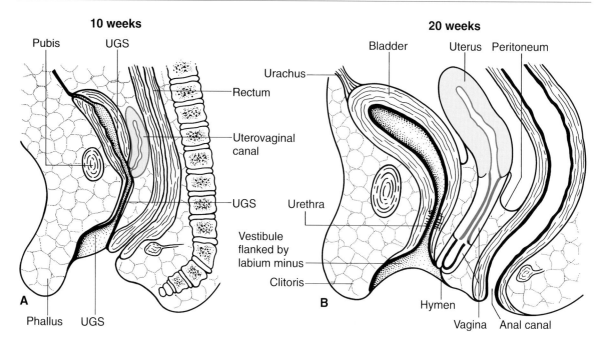

Figure 23.4. Female pelvic organs in sagittal section. The paramesonephric epithelial lining of the vagina is shown in blue, the sinual (UGS) lining in black. UGS, urogenital sinus.

At first, the urethra opens on the under surface of the phallus, proximal to an expansion formed by the developing **glans**. During the 4th month an ectodermal invagination grows in from the tip of the glans to form the **glandar urethra**, whereupon the proximal opening is sealed off.

The **prepuce** is a collar-like outgrowth of skin from the base of the glans.

The genital swellings enlarge to form the two halves of the **scrotum**. They come together below the bulb of the urethra. The line of union of the two scrotal swellings is marked by a **scrotal raphe**.

Female External Genitalia (Figure 23.5D,E)

The female external genitalia arise by the continued growth *in situ* of the urogenital folds and genital swellings. The phallus forms the **clitoris**, tipped by a small glans.

The urethral groove and the phallic part of the urogenital sinus remain open as the **vestibule**. The urogenital folds become the labia minora flanking the vestibule, and the genital swellings become the **labia majora**. The labia majora come together between anus and vestibule, in the **caudal (posterior) commissure**.

ANAL CANAL

The mature anal canal is the part of the alimentary tract that lies below the level of the levator ani muscle (*Figure 23.3*). The upper half of the canal is lined by columnar, endodermal epithelium continuous with that of the rectum. The lower half develops from the anal pit and is lined by stratified squamous epithelium continuous with the epidermis of the surrounding skin.

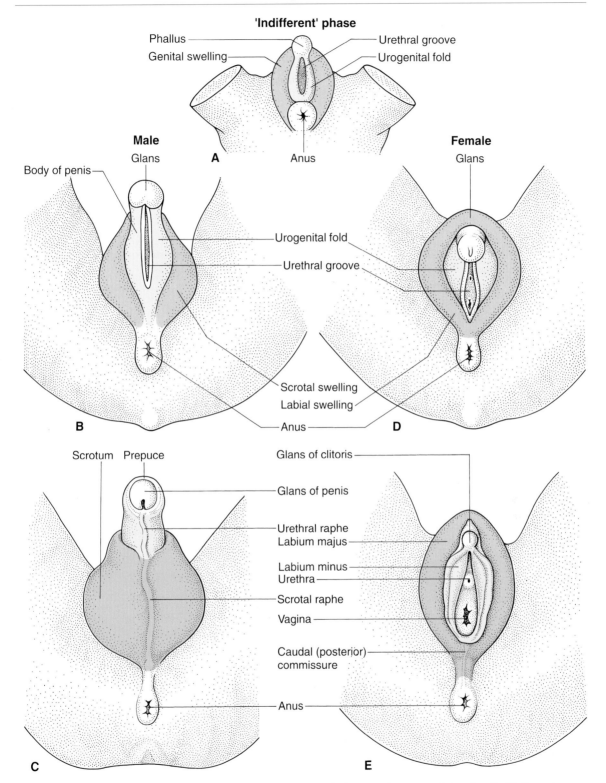

Figure 23.5. Development of external genitalia. (A) Indifferent phase. (B,C) Male. (D,E) Female.

MALFORMATIONS

Bladder and Urethra

In *hypospadias*, which occurs in 0.2% of males, there is an opening in the floor of the urethra, and the normal external meatus is absent. In accordance with the position of the abnormal opening, hypospadias is described as *glandar, penile, scrotal* or *perineal*.

In *phimosis*, the opening of the collar-like prepuce is so fine that it obstructs the outflow of urine during micturition. Manual retraction of a narrow prepuce may result in compression of the spongy urethra (*paraphimosis*).

External Genitalia

A *true hermaphrodite* is an individual who possesses functional testicular and ovarian tissue, either in the same gonad or in opposite gonads. The condition is extremely rare. A uterus and a vagina are present. The external genitalia may be either male or female in type.

A *pseudohermaphrodite* is an individual whose genotypic sex is at variance with the phenotypic sex, i.e. with the sexual anatomy. *Female* pseudohermaphrodites are of female genotype and have male features such as enlargement of the clitoris and more or less complete fusion of the labia majora. The explanation nearly always lies in an *adrenogenital syndrome* brought about by congenital hyperplasia of the suprarenal cortex. In this condition there is an enzyme defect on the pathway to the synthesis of cortisol; instead of cortisol, other steroids are produced, some having androgenic influence upon the external genitalia. *Male* pseudohermaphrodites are of male genotype with a female phenotype, e.g. with undescended testes and a scrotal hypospadias. The cause may lie in deficient testosterone production or deficient target-cell sensitivity to testosterone.

Anal Canal and Rectum

Failure to pass meconium within 24 hours after birth leads to suspicion of large bowel obstruction. The commonest cause is *Hirschsprung's disease*, where the rectum and sigmoid colon are in a state of tonic spasm, due to absence of autonomic ganglion cells ('aganglionic segment' of the gut). The reason may lie in failure of neuroblasts to migrate from the neural crest to the hindgut, or in failure of the gut to sustain them after their arrival. The second explanation seems more likely, since ganglion cells usually succeed in seeding the wall of the bladder. Hirschsprung's disease results in progressive accumulation of colonic contents, with distension of the abdomen.

Other causes of large bowel obstruction fall under the general heading, *anorectal agenesis*. In some cases, the anal canal is absent, and the rectum opens into the bladder (in males) or vagina. In others, the anal canal is separated from the rectum by a thin tissue diaphragm (*imperforate anus*).

EMBRYOLOGICAL TERMS

Genital tubercle. Urorectal septum. Phallus. Urogenital sinus. Urogenital membrane. Anal membrane. Anal pit. Primitive bladder. Sinual tubercle (Müllerian eminence). Vaginal plate. Urethral groove. Urogenital folds. Genital swellings. *Hypospadias. Phimosis. Paraphimosis. Hermaphrodite. Pseudohermaphrodite. Hirschsprung's disease. Anorectal agenesis. Imperforate anus.*

24

Head and neck: pharyngeal arches, pouches and clefts

PHARYNGEAL ARCHES

Figure 24.1 represents a side view of the rostral part of an embryo late in the 5th week. The pharyngeal arches are numbered I, II, III, IV and VI. (In higher mammals, the fifth arches are no more than transient.) The arches are composed of mesoderm.

Phylogenetically, the pharyngeal arches are homologous with the gill arches (*branchia*) of fishes. However, the gill slits present in fishes do not appear in mammals, where successive arches remain linked by the mesoderm.

Placodes of the Head and Neck

A number of localized thickenings of the surface ectoderm, the *placodes*, are shown in *Figure 24.1*. Three of them have been mentioned in previous chapters, namely the nasal placode, the lens placode, and the otic placode. The last named recedes beneath the surface during the 4th week and becomes the *otocyst*. Four further, *epibranchial placodes* contribute sensory ganglion cells to underlying cranial nerves.

Sources of Mesoderm in the Head and Neck

The mesoderm of the head and neck originates almost entirely from two sources: the paraxial mesoderm and the neural crest (*Figure 24.2A*).

Paraxial Mesoderm

The paraxial mesoderm is divisible into three parts:

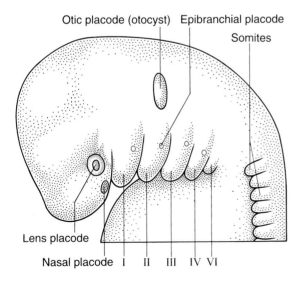

Otic placode (otocyst) Epibranchial placode

Somites

Lens placode

Nasal placode I   II   III IV VI

Figure 24.1. Left side of a 5-week embryo.

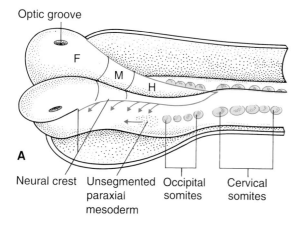

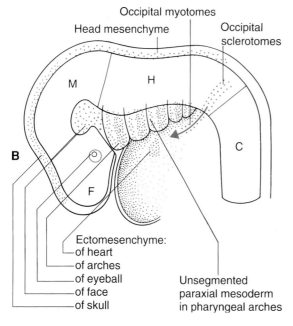

Figure 24.2. Sources of pharyngeal arch mesoderm. (A) Dorsal view of 24-day embryo. Arrows indicate directions of migrations. (B) Side view during 5th week. F, forebrain; M, midbrain; H, hindbrain; C, spinal cord.

- The most rostral part does not undergo segmentation to form somites. Instead, this *parachordal mesoderm* migrates widely, forming the bulk of the pharyngeal arch mesoderm, and of the *head mesenchyme* investing the brain (*Figure 24.2B*).
- The first four, occipital somites separate into sclerotomes that contribute to the occipital bone, myotomes that form the muscles of the tongue (Figure 24.2B), and dermatomes that form the dermis of the skin in the occipital region.
- The eight pairs of cervical somites separate into sclerotomes that form the cervical vertebral column, myotomes that form the segmentally innervated muscles of the neck, and dermatomes that form the dermis of the neck.

Neural Crest

The neural crest is the ribbon of cells that detaches from the neural folds during closure of the neural tube. It extends rostrally along the margins of the brain plate (*Figure 24.2A*). Some cells of neural crest origin, called *ectomesenchyme*, have the capacity to form tissues which in other areas are produced by the mesoderm. The distribution of migrant ectomesenchymal cells is as follows (*Figure 24.2B*):

- From the hindbrain, they enter the pharyngeal arches and become cartilage and bone-forming cells within each one. Some cells leave the arches and form the wall of the outflow channel of the heart (Chapter 16).
- From the midbrain, they contribute to the skeleton and connective tissue of the face, and to the teeth (Chapter 26).
- From the forebrain, they contribute to the vascular and fibrous coats of the eyeball (Chapter 28).

Common Features of the Pharyngeal Arches (Figure 24.3)
Every arch contains the following structures:

- A core of cartilage derived from neural crest cells.
- Unsegmented mesoderm capable of forming striated muscle and bone.

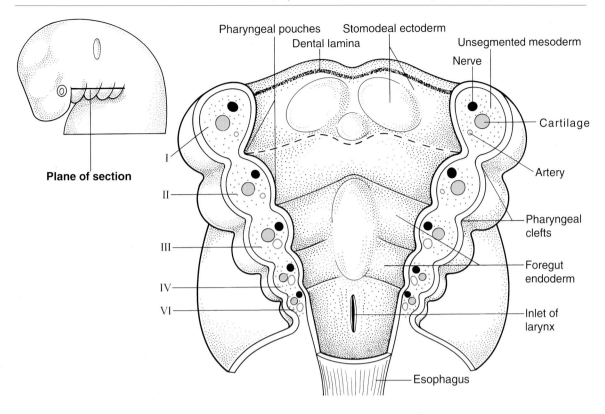

Figure 24.3. Transverse section through the pharyngeal arches, to show their contents. Dashed line represents the former site of attachment of the oral membrane.

- An artery that runs from the aortic sac to the dorsal aorta on the same side.
- A nerve that enters it from the brain stem. The nerve carries motor fibers called *special visceral (branchial) efferents*, for the supply of striated muscles developing from the unsegmented mesoderm.

The inner and outer surfaces of the arches have epithelial linings that enter pockets in the interval between successive arches. The internal pockets are called *pharyngeal pouches*, the external ones being *pharyngeal clefts*.

The development of the individual pharyngeal arches will now be considered in turn.

First Pharyngeal Arch

The first pair of pharyngeal arches, the *mandibular* arches, come together in the floor of the stomodeum (*Figures 24.4* and *24.5*). A *maxillary prominence* arises from the dorsal part of each, lateral to the stomodeum. During the 5th week, the two maxillary prominences meet one another above the stomodeum and collaborate in forming the palate (see later).

In the core of the mandibular arch, ectomesenchymal cells form *Meckel's cartilage*, which serves as a template for development of the mandible (*Figure 24.4*). During the 6th and later weeks, membrane bone is laid down (also by ectomesenchyme) on the

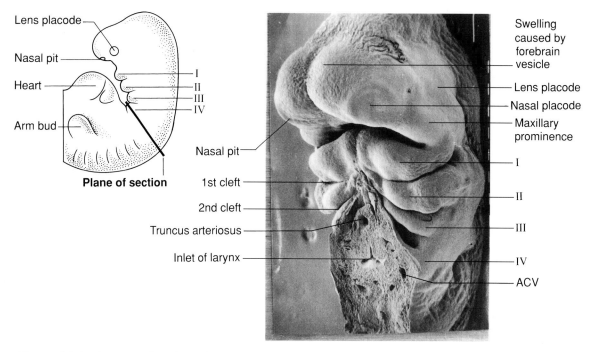

Figure 24.4. Pharyngeal arches of a 33-day embryo. The nasal pit is shallower than is usual at this age. ACV, anterior cardinal vein. (From a photograph kindly provided by Professor S. Viragh, Postgraduate Medical School, Budapest.)

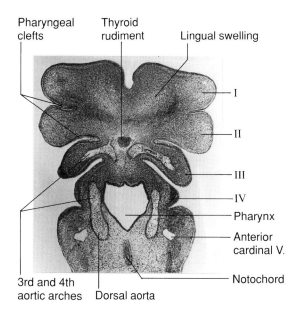

Figure 24.5. Tangential section taken through the pharyngeal arches, at 5 weeks. (Carnegie Collection.)

outer surface of the cartilage, forming the mandible proper.

The dorsal end of Meckel's cartilage is incorporated into the middle ear, where it forms the **malleus** and the **incus**. In the interval between ear and mandible, the perichondrium alone persists, as the **sphenomandibular ligament** (*Figure 24.6*).

Ectomesenchyme contained in the maxillary prominence gives rise to the **maxilla**, the **zygomatic bone**, and the **squamous temporal bone**, by a means of intramembranous ossification (*Figure 24.6*).

The muscles formed from mandibular arch mesoderm are the **muscles of mastication**, namely the masseter, temporalis, pterygoids, anterior digastric and mylohyoid. The tensor tympani and tensor palati muscles are also of mandibular arch origin.

The branchial efferent nerve supply to all of these muscles is the **mandibular branch of the trigeminal nerve**.

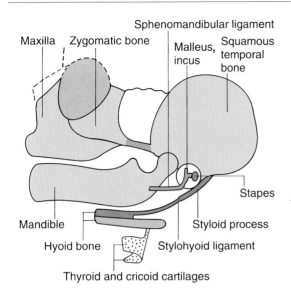

Figure 24.6. Full-term skull, showing skeletal derivatives of pharyngeal arches. Arches: I, red; II, black; III, blue; IV and VI, stipple.

Mandibular arch ectomesenchyme forms the connective tissue of the skin and mucous membranes of the face and mouth. They receive a somatic sensory nerve supply from the **ophthalmic, maxillary and mandibular branches of the trigeminal nerve.**

Second Pharyngeal Arch

The second or *hyoid arch* has a smaller skeletal component than the first. No membrane bone forms from it. The hyoid arch cartilage undergoes endochondral ossification at its dorsal end to form the **incus** and the **stapes**, and at its ventral end to form the **upper part of the hyoid bone** (*Figure 24.6*). The perichondrium of this arch persists in the interval between ear and hyoid bone, as the **stylohyoid ligament**.

Most of the mesoderm of the second arch migrates over the surface of the face, skull and neck. The migratory mesoderm forms the **muscles of facial expression**, which are characterized by their insertion into the skin – unlike the masticatory muscles, which insert into the mandible. Additional muscles formed from hyoid arch mesoderm are the **posterior digastric**, **stapedius** and **stylohyoid**.

The **facial nerve** carries the branchial efferent nerve supply to the hyoid arch musculature. It also carries sensory fibers that supply taste buds in the anterior part of the tongue (*Figure 24.7*).

Third Pharyngeal Arch

The third arch forms the primordium of the posterior part of the **tongue** (see later). The cartilage of this arch provides the **lower half of the hyoid bone**. The only muscle formed from the arch is the **stylopharyngeus**.

The **glossopharyngeal nerve** carries the branchial efferent nerve supply to the stylopharyngeus. It also carries general sense and taste fibers serving the posterior part of the tongue.

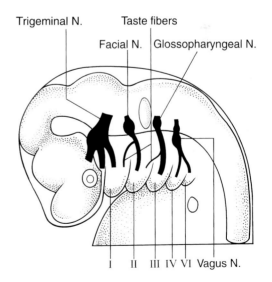

Figure 24.7. Nerve supply of the pharyngeal arches.

The artery of the third arch persists as the proximal part of the **internal carotid artery** (*Figure 24.8*).

Fourth and Sixth Pharyngeal Arches

The fourth and sixth arches come together to yield the **cartilages and ligaments of the larynx**, the **intrinsic muscles of the larynx** and the **levator palati**. The nerve of supply is the **vagus**, through its laryngeal and pharyngeal branches. The motor fibers in these nerves originate in the nucleus ambiguus in the medulla oblongata; they enter the vagus via the cranial accessory nerve (see Chapter 30).

The histories of the arteries of the fourth and sixth arches are given in Chapter 13. In summary, the left fourth arch artery contributes to the arch of the aorta; the right one forms most of the right subclavian artery.

THE TONGUE

The primordium of the anterior part of the tongue arises from the first pharyngeal arch. The second arch mesoderm migrates away from the floor of the foregut, and the third and fourth arches provide the primordium for the posterior part of the tongue. The lingual musculature is derived from occipital myotomes.

The anterior part of the tongue consists initially of paired *lateral lingual swellings* flanking a single *median lingual swelling* (*Figure 24.9A*). These three coalesce to form the mesenchymal primordium of the anterior two-thirds of the tongue. The primordium of the posterior one-third originates from a single swelling, the *hypopharyngeal eminence*, belonging to the third and fourth arches.

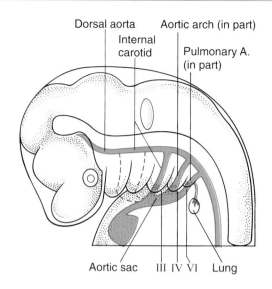

Figure 24.8. Pharyngeal arch arteries.

Following migration of the hyoid arch mesoderm to form the muscles of facial expression (*Figure 24.9B*), the posterior and anterior elements come together. Their junction is marked by the V-shaped **sulcus terminalis** on each side, and by the **foramen cecum** in the midline (*Figure 24.9C*).

The mucous membrane of the anterior two-thirds of the tongue is supplied by the lingual branch of the mandibular nerve. The glossopharyngeal nerve is sensory to most of the posterior one-third, also to the circumvallate papillae (taste) directly anterior to the sulcus terminalis. The mucous membrane over the root of the tongue is supplied by the superior laryngeal branch of the vagus nerve.

The mesenchymal primordia of the tongue provide a scaffolding for the migration of myoblasts originating in the occipital myotomes. The myoblasts form the intrinsic and extrinsic muscles of the tongue. Because it is derived from myotomes, the lingual musculature is of somite rather than branchial origin. It is supplied by the **hypoglossal nerve**, whose nucleus is in line with the somatic efferent cell column of the

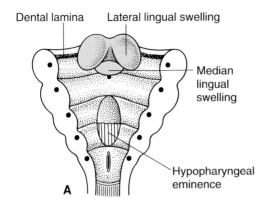

Dental lamina   Lateral lingual swelling

Median lingual swelling

Hypopharyngeal eminence

A

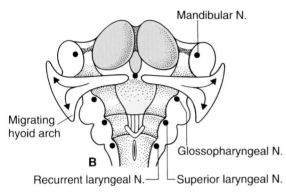

Mandibular N.

Migrating hyoid arch

Glossopharyngeal N.

B

Recurrent laryngeal N.   Superior laryngeal N.

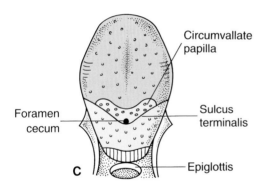

Circumvallate papilla

Foramen cecum

Sulcus terminalis

Epiglottis

C

Figure 24.9. Development of the tongue.

spinal cord. (A single exception is the palatoglossus, which is supplied by the pharyngeal branch of the vagus.)

DERIVATIVES OF THE PHARYNGEAL POUCHES

The pharyngeal pouches are the endodermal pockets on each side of the pharynx, in the intervals between successive pharyngeal arches (*Figure 24.10*). The first four pouches are well defined, the fifth poorly.

First Pharyngeal Pouch

The dorsal part of the first pouch gives rise to the *tubotympanic recess*, which is the primordium of the **auditory (Eustachian) tube** and the **middle ear cavity**. (See The ear, in Chapter 27.)

Second Pharyngeal Pouch

The epithelium in the ventral part of the second pouch thickens and sends buds into the underlying mesenchyme, forming the primordium of the **tonsil**. The mesenchyme becomes seeded with lymphocytes which multiply to form lymphatic nodules, thereby establishing the definitive tonsil. The **intratonsillar cleft** in the upper part of

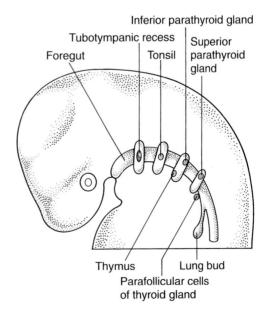

Inferior parathyroid gland

Tubotympanic recess   Superior parathyroid gland

Foregut   Tonsil

Thymus   Lung bud

Parafollicular cells of thyroid gland

Figure 24.10. Pharyngeal pouches and their derivatives.

the adult gland is a remnant of the second pouch.

Third Pharyngeal Pouch

The **thymus** is a bilobed gland that arises bilaterally from the ventral part of the third pouch. The two lobes come into contact with the aortic sac, which draws the gland into the superior mediastinum during the descent of the heart. The original endodermal buds give rise to the thymic reticular cells. The interstices of the reticulum are seeded by cells which develop into immunologically competent T lymphocytes; these are exported by the thymus to the other lymphoid tissues via the blood stream.

The thymus reaches its maximum *relative* size at full term, in relation to the body weight (*Figure 24.11*). It reaches its maximum *absolute* size at puberty, then undergoes regression.

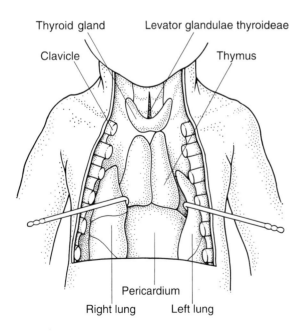

Figure 24.11. Thyroid and thymus glands at full term.

The **inferior parathyroid gland** arises from endoderm in the dorsal part of the third pouch on each side. It descends along with the thymus and then leaves it to become embedded in the back of the thyroid gland. It is not unusual for the inferior parathyroid to follow the thymus into the superior mediastinum.

Fourth Pharyngeal Pouch

The **superior parathyroid gland** arises from endoderm in the dorsal part of the fourth pouch on each side. It becomes embedded in the back of the thyroid gland without undergoing significant descent.

Fifth Pharyngeal Pouch

The **parafollicular, C cells of the thyroid gland**, which secrete calcitonin, originate from neural crest cells that have migrated to the endoderm of the fifth pouch.

The **glomus cells** of the carotid and aortic bodies are also of neural crest origin. They probably travel by way of the fifth pouch.

THYROID GLAND

The thyroid gland arises as a *median thyroid rudiment* from midline pharyngeal endoderm (*Figure 24.5*). The point of origin is marked permanently by the **foramen cecum** at the apex of the sulcus terminalis (*Figure 24.9C*). The median thyroid rudiment sinks into the mesoderm overlying the aortic sac, and descends in company with the thymus and the inferior parathyroid glands. The path taken by the thyroid is marked for a time by the *thyroglossal duct*, a cord of cells linking the gland to the foramen cecum.

The median rudiment bifurcates to form two **lobes**, connected to one another by an **isthmus**. The position of the lower part of the thyroglossal duct may be permanently represented by a **pyramidal lobe**, or by some smooth muscle, the **levator glandulae thyroideae**, projecting upward from the isthmus (*Figure 24.11*).

DERIVATIVES OF THE PHARYNGEAL CLEFTS

Only the first cleft is normally of permanent significance. It gives rise to the **external acoustic meatus**. (See The ear, in Chapter 27.)

When the second pharyngeal arch extends down the neck to create the platysma muscle sheet, it fuses below with a mesodermal *epipericardial ridge* containing the anterior cardinal vein. Some of the surface ectoderm becomes trapped in a cystic space, the *cervical sinus*, which is normally obliterated.

MALFORMATIONS

Thyroid Gland

Congenital hypothyroidism occurs in 1 in 3000 live births. It is a significant cause of mental handicap, because maturation of neurons in the cerebral cortex depends upon an adequate supply of hormones T3 and T4. During fetal life, neuronal development may be adequate because of hormonal transfer across the placenta. In neonates, the clinician may be alerted by the physical appearance and behavior: coarseness of facial appearance, hoarseness, dry skin, floppy limbs, constipation. Raised TSH (thyroid-stimulating hormone) levels in the blood indicate urgent need for medication with thyroxine.

Errors of Thyroid Descent

Very rarely, the thyroid rudiment may fail to descend from its point of origin. Instead, it enlarges *in situ* as a *lingual thyroid gland* which projects into the oropharynx and may obstruct it.

Persistence of part or all of the thyroglossal duct is more common. The usual presentation takes the form of a *thyroglossal cyst* during childhood or later. Diagnostic features are: (a) a midline presentation in the lower part of the neck, and (b) movement of the cyst on swallowing, because of duct remnants anchoring it to the hyoid bone. A cyst may break down, creating a *thyroglossal fistula* in the midline.

Branchial Cyst

A remnant of the cervical sinus may present itself as a *branchial cyst* during childhood or later life. A branchial cyst is characteristically soft to the touch, usually presenting at the anterior border of the sternomastoid below the angle of the jaw. The cyst may break down to create a fistula.

EMBRYOLOGICAL TERMS

Pharyngeal arches. Epibranchial placodes. Special visceral efferent nerves. Pharyngeal pouches. Pharyngeal clefts. Mandibular arch. Maxillary prominence. Meckel's cartilage. Hyoid arch. Lingual swellings. Hypopharyngeal eminence. Tubotympanic recess. Median thyroid rudiment. Cervical sinus. *Congenital hypothyroidism. Lingual thyroid. Thyroglossal cyst/fistula. Branchial cyst/fistula.*

25

Head and neck: face and palate

FACE

Facial Prominences

Mesoderm that forms the embryonic connective tissue framework of the face is ectomesenchyme derived from the neural crest. In the region of the future face, the mesoderm produces five elevations called *prominences* that merge with one another under cover of the surface ectoderm. Movement of the facial mesoderm commences early in the 5th week. It is largely concluded 3 weeks later. The disposition of the young connective cells and fibers serves to guide the premuscle cells of the mandibular and hyoid arches toward appropriate bony attachments.

Figure 25.1A–D illustrates successive stages in the development of the face. Early in the 5th week (*Figure 25.1A*), the nasal placodes are receding into the nasal pits. The lens placodes lie above the maxillary prominences. The mesoderm over the bulging forebrain vesicle is thickening to form the *frontonasal prominence*.

Early in the 6th week (*Figure 25.1B*), the frontonasal prominence extends onto both sides of each nasal pit, creating *medial and lateral nasal prominences*. The nasal pits become deep, *nasal sacs*, opening to the surface through *anterior nares* (the **nostrils**).

During the 5th and 6th weeks, the mandibular arches share in the formation of the lower jaw and the connective tissue of the lower lip. On the side of the neck, mandibular and hyoid mesoderm are forming *aural hillocks*, which in due course form the auricle of the ear (see Chapter 27).

Late in the 6th week (*Figure 25.1C*), mesoderm of frontonasal origin is marked off from the maxillary prominence by a *nasolacrimal furrow*. In the midline, frontonasal mesoderm forms the bridge of the nose.

The surface ectoderm in the nasolacrimal furrow forms a cord of cells which sinks into the mesoderm and becomes canalized. The outer end of the canal forms the **lacrimal sac**. The inner end opens into the floor of the nostril, completing the **nasolacrimal duct**.

Intermaxillary Segment

The two medial nasal prominences merge across the midline, creating a rectangular block of mesoderm known as the *intermaxillary segment*.

During the 7th week (*Figure 25.1D*), the intermaxillary segment produces three midline structures: (a) the lower border of the **nasal septum**; (b) the **philtrum** of the upper lip; and under cover of the philtrum, (c) the *primary palate*, which is the forerunner of the premaxilla. (Some workers maintain that the philtrum is formed by an overgrowth of maxillary mesoderm.)

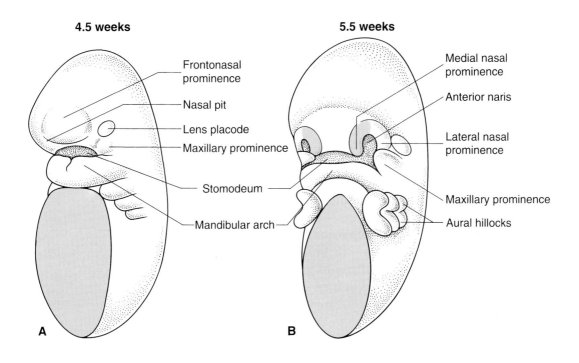

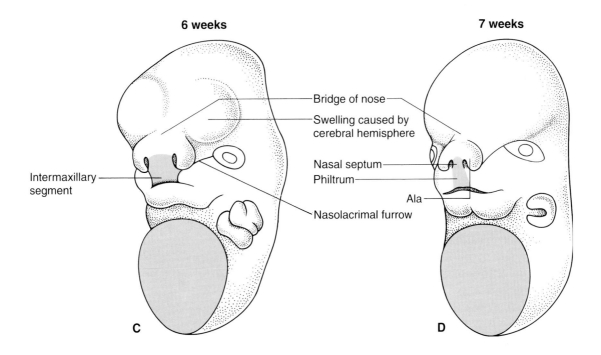

Figure 25.1. Development of the face. Medial nasal processes and intermaxillary segment are shown in red.

The mesodermal elements of the face are increased by the arrival of a wave of hyoid arch mesoderm which differentiates into the muscles of facial expression. Masticatory muscles developing from mandibular arch mesoderm extend onto the side of the face (masseter) and skull (temporalis).

The lateral nasal prominence on each side creates the **ala** (wing) of the nose. Maxillary mesoderm merges with this prominence, superficial to the nasolacrimal duct.

Intramembranous ossification within the maxillary mesoderm produces, from before backward, the **maxilla**, the **zygomatic bone**, and the **squamous temporal bone** (see *Figure 24.6*). The two **nasal bones** in the bridge of the nose, and the **vomer** in the nasal septum develop from frontonasal mesoderm.

PALATE

Major features of palatal development are viewed from below in *Figure 25.2A-C*. During the 7th week (*Figure 25.2A*), the floor of the nasal sac gives way, creating the *primitive posterior naris*. At the same time, mesoderm of the intermaxillary segment extends backward in the midline, as a blunt *nasal septum*. *Palatal shelves*, which originated from the maxillary prominence a week earlier, extend into the oral cavity and hang down on either side of the tongue.

Two curved bands of thickened ectoderm appear in the roof of the stomodeum; a matching two appear in its floor. The inner one of each pair, the *dental lamina*, gives rise to ten *tooth buds* for the deciduous dentition (see Chapter 26). The other one, the *vestibular lamina*, excavates the underlying mesoderm to create the **vestibule**, i.e. the trough that separates the teeth from the lip and cheek.

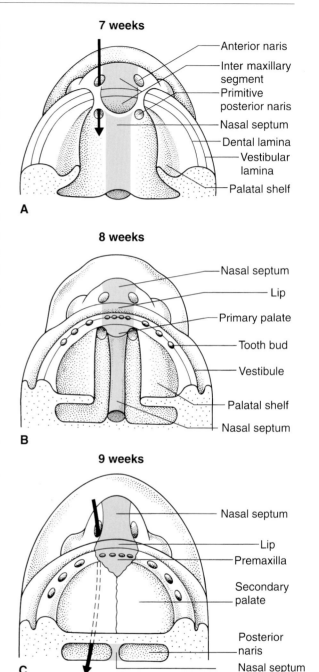

Figure 25.2. Head region, viewed from below, showing development of the palate. In (A) and (C), an arrow is passing along the nasal passage on one side.

Primary and Secondary Palate

During the 8th week (*Figure 25.2B*), the intermaxillary segment separates into three parts: the free edge of the nasal septum, in front; the philtrum of the upper lip, in the middle; and the *primary palate*, behind.

During the same week, the mandibular arches have become wide enough to allow the tongue to descend from its position between the palatal shelves. Thus freed, the shelves move into a horizontal position within a matter of hours. They grow across the upper surface of the tongue and, during the 9th or 10th week, they fuse with the primary palate and then with one another (*Figure 25.2C*). This completes the *secondary palate*.

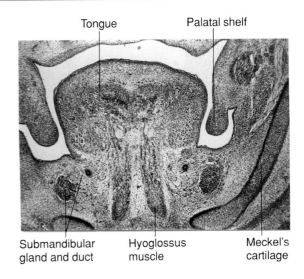

Tongue   Palatal shelf

Submandibular gland and duct   Hyoglossus muscle   Meckel's cartilage

Figure 25.3. Frontal section through the oral region, early in the 8th week. (Cambridge Collection.)

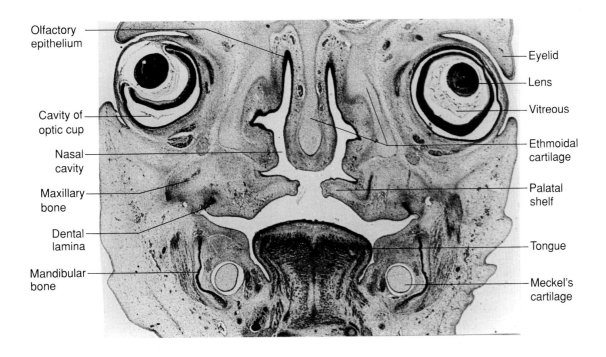

Olfactory epithelium

Cavity of optic cup

Nasal cavity

Maxillary bone

Dental lamina

Mandibular bone

Eyelid

Lens

Vitreous

Ethmoidal cartilage

Palatal shelf

Tongue

Meckel's cartilage

Figure 25.4. Frontal section through face and oral region, at 8 weeks. (Cambridge Collection.)

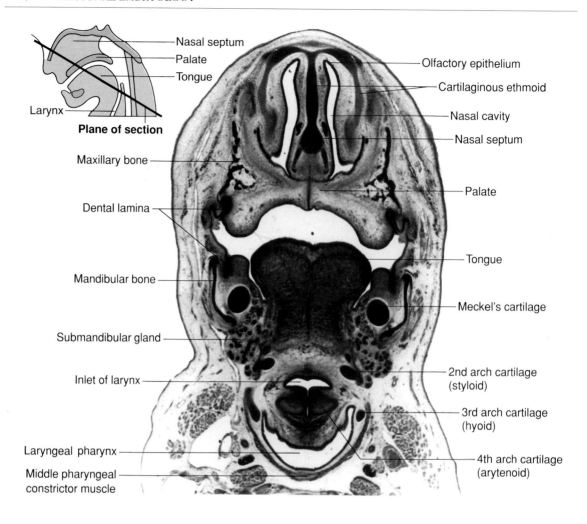

Figure 25.5. Frontal section through splanchnocranium and neck, at 11 weeks. (Carnegie Collection.)

Nasal Cavity, Definitive Palate

The height of the nasal septum increases by the upward extension of the nasal sac on either side of it. The skeleton of the septum receives contributions from the *nasal capsule* (see Chapter 26). The septum fuses with the upper surface of the secondary palate. The **nasal cavities** now extend along the upper surface of the palate on each side of the septum, opening into the pharynx at the **definitive posterior nares (posterior nasal apertures)** (*Figure 25.2C*).

The three developmental levels illustrated in *Figure 25.2*, are shown in coronal sections in *Figures 25.3, 25.4* and *25.5*.

The **definitive palate** is established by intramembranous ossification anteriorly (creating the hard palate) and by the entry of myoblasts posteriorly (creating the soft palate). The myoblasts enter from first and fourth arch mesoderm (to form the tensor and levator palati muscles, respectively).

MALFORMATIONS

Cleft lip and *cleft palate* are among the commoner congenital malformations. They occur, singly or together, once in about 800 births. Genetic or environmental factors may predominate in a particular case.

Cleft lip is commoner in boys. The cleft extends from the anterior naris to the mouth. In severe cases there is a cleft upper jaw as well, reaching as far back as the incisive foramen and separating the primary from the secondary palate on that side.

Cleft palate is commoner in girls. The mildest cleft gives rise only to a bifid uvula; moderate cases show cleavage of the soft palate; and severe cases show complete cleavage of the soft and hard palate. Most severe of all is a combination of a complete cleft palate with a cleft upper jaw and lip on both sides; here the premaxilla is attached only to the nasal septum.

EMBRYOLOGICAL TERMS

Frontonasal prominence. Lateral and medial nasal prominences. Nasal pit. Nasal sac. Aural hillocks. Nasolacrimal furrow. Intermaxillary segment. Primary palate. Primitive posterior naris. Palatal shelves. Secondary palate. *Cleft lip. Cleft palate.*

26

Head and neck: skull and teeth, salivary glands

SKULL

Adult Anatomy

The adult skull (cranium) is made up of neurocranium and viscerocranium, as follows:

The **neurocranium** is the bony case enclosing the brain. It comprises the **base** and the **vault (calvaria)** of the skull. The base contains the **chondrocranium** (cartilaginous cranium), derived from endochondral ossification of the heavier parts of the occipital, temporal and sphenoid bones and of the entire ethmoid bone. The vault consists of membrane bones (the frontal and parietal bones and the outermost parts of the occipital, temporal and sphenoid bones).

The **viscerocranium** is the skeleton of the face; it consists of membrane bones including the mandible, the maxillae, the nasal and zygomatic bones, and the vomer. The frontal bone also contributes.

Development

Several lines of evidence indicate that the bones of the chondrocranium and viscerocranium develop mainly from ectomesoderm of neural crest origin. The vault develops from paraxial mesoderm.

Chondrocranium (Figure 26.1)

The chondrocranium develops from eight pairs of cartilaginous precursors (*Figure 26.1A*). Four pairs are close to the midline, as follows:

- *Occipital sclerotomes*, derived from the occipital somites.
- *Parachordal cartilages*, derived from the parachordal mesoderm.
- *Hypophyseal cartilages*, beside the pituitary gland.
- *Prechordal cartilages*, rostral to the pituitary gland.

Each of the other four pairs develops in relation to special senses, as follows:

- The *otic capsule* encloses the inner ear.
- The *alisphenoid* and *orbitosphenoid* enclose the back of the eye.
- The *nasal capsule* encloses the olfactory epithelium

Development of the individual skull bones can be followed in *Figure 26.1B and C*.

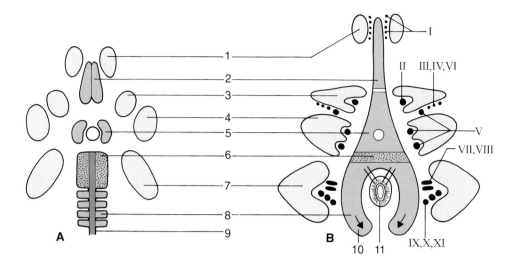

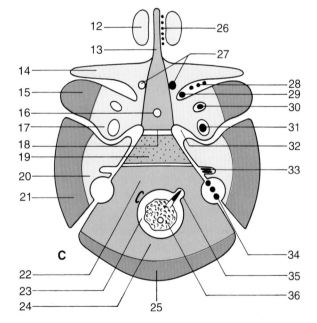

1. Nasal capsule
2. Prechordal cartilages
3. Orbitosphenoid
4. Alisphenoid
5. Hypophysial cartilage
6. Parachordal cartilage
7. Otic capsule
8. Occipital somites
9. Notochord
10 Neural arch
11. Neural tube
12. Ethmoidal labyrinth
13. Crista galli, perpendicular plate of
     ethmoid
14. Lesser wing of sphenoid bone
15. Greater wing of sphenoid bone, outer part
16. Hypophysial fossa in body of
     sphenoid bone
17. Greater wing of sphenoid bone, inner part
18. Spheno-occipital synchondrosis
19. Anterior component of basiocciput
20. Petromastoid cartilage
21. Squamous temporal bone
22. Posterior component of basiocciput
23. Foramen magnum
24. Postoccipital cartilage
25. Interparietal part of occipital bone
26. Olfactory nerve bundles
27. Optic nerve and canal
28. Nerves III, IV and VI in superior
     orbital fissure

29. Ophthalmic V
30. Maxillary V in foramen rotundum
31. Mandibular V in foramen ovale
32. Foramen lacerum
33. VII and VIII in internal acoustic meatus
34. IX, X, XI in jugular foramen
35. XII in hypoglossal canal
36. Medulla oblongata

Figure 26.1. Diagrams showing components of developing skull. Endochondral bone, blue; membrane bone, red.

- *Occipital bone.* The parachordal mesoderm and occipital sclerotomes merge to form the primordium of the basiocciput. Prior to chondrification, the sclerotomes send neural arches around the junction of spinal cord and brain stem, creating the postocciput. The interparietal part of the occipital bone belongs to the vault of the skull and ossifies in membrane.
- *Sphenoid bone.* The hypophysial cartilages form the body of the sphenoid and enclose the hypophysial fossa. The orbitosphenoid cartilage forms the lesser wing of the sphenoid. The inner part of the greater wing also belongs to the skull base and ossifies from the alisphenoid cartilage. The outer part of the greater wing belongs to the vault and ossifies in membrane.
- *Temporal bone.* There are four parts to the temporal bone. The petromastoid part develops from the cartilaginous *otic capsule* surrounding the membranous labyrinth. (The mastoid element appears postnatally.) The styloid process ossifies from second pharyngeal arch cartilage. The squamous temporal belongs to the skull vault and ossifies in membrane. Finally, the tympanic plate (in the floor of the external acoustic meatus) also ossifies in membrane.
- *Ethmoid bone.* The prechordal cartilages are included in the crista galli and perpendicular plate. The lateral masses (labyrinths) develop from the cartilaginous nasal capsules.

The relationships of the basal cartilages to the cranial nerves, and the major cranial foramina, are also shown in *Figure 26.1*.

Ossification of the chondrocranium takes place from multiple centers, most of them appearing between the 8th and 16th weeks. Following ossification of the basilar parts of the occipital and sphenoid bones, continued elongation of the cranial base in prenatal and postnatal life originates at the **spheno-occipital synchondrosis**, a primary cartilaginous joint.

Vault

The skull vault undergoes intramembranous ossification from the 3rd month onward. Separate ossification centers give rise to the parietal bone, the outer part of the greater wing of the sphenoid bone, the squamous part of the temporal bone, and the interparietal part of the occipital bone. The frontal bone develops from two separate centers, in the region of the future frontal eminences. Plates of bone derived from the two centers are quite separate at first, and they produce their own orbital plates. The plates blend across the midline later on, but fusion is not completed until the 8th postnatal year.

In the newborn skull, the **frontal and parietal eminences** are pronounced (*Figure 26.2*). They mark the sites of the respective centers of ossification. The **anterior fontanelle** is a diamond-shaped, fibrous mesodermal sheet bounded by the frontal and parietal bones. It is clinically of great importance for the assessment of the state of hydration, being sunken in dehydrated infants. It is palpable for 18 months after birth and is closed off by sutural contact 6 months later. A triangular **posterior fontanelle** between the parietal and occipital bones, closes 2 months after birth.

Viscerocranium

All of the facial bones ossify in membrane from neural crest elements contained in the frontonasal and maxillary prominences and in the mandibular arch. The bones concerned are the nasal and lacrimal, the maxillary and zygomatic, and the vomer.

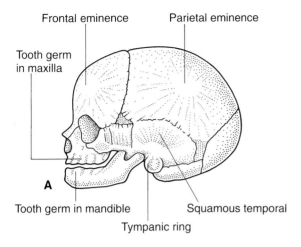

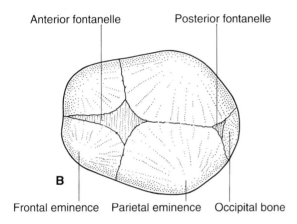

Figure 26.2. The skull at birth. (A) From the left side. (B) From above.

The *mandible* is the first skeletal element in the body to commence ossification; a single center appears on each side, lateral to Meckel's cartilage early in the 6th week. The cartilage serves as a template around which membrane bone is laid down to form the **body** of the mandible. The **ramus** develops by *endochondral ossification* from a *condylar growth center* that makes its appearance in the 14th week. The center is formed by cartilaginous transformation of mandibular arch mesenchyme, in the region of the future condyle. Additional cells are added to the cartilaginous condyle from the perichondrium covering its upper surface. The carti-

lage itself behaves in the manner of an epiphysial plate, paying out cell columns which become calcified and then ossified. The condylar growth center is responsible for elongation of the ramus during the first 10 years of postnatal life.

TEETH

Tooth Buds, Enamel Organs, Tooth Germs

Figure 26.3A–C contains diagrams of the mandibular arch, representing important early steps in development of the teeth. In *Figure 26.3A*, the dental lamina is a curved band of thickened ectoderm. In *Figure 26.3B*, ten tooth buds are formed from the dental lamina – five on each side. In addition, the vestibular lamina is a second, parallel band, external to the dental lamina. In *Figure 26.3C*, the vestibular lamina has

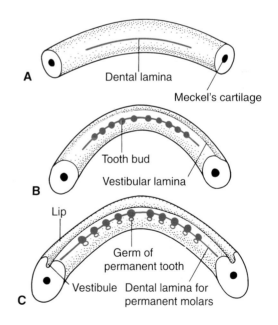

Figure 26.3. Diagrams showing features of dental development in the lower jaw.

excavated the mesoderm, thereby creating the vestibule.

The ten tooth buds are responsible for the development of the deciduous dentition, which comprises two incisor teeth, one canine tooth, and two molar teeth on each side. The entire deciduous dentition therefore consists of 20 teeth. Later (*Figure 26.3C*), the dental lamina goes on to form the buds of the permanent teeth that replace the deciduous set – namely, two permanent incisors, one canine and two *premolars*. The three permanent molar teeth are without any deciduous precursors. They develop postnatally, from a backward extension of the dental lamina (*Figure 26.3C*).

Early steps in development of a mandibular incisor tooth are shown in *Figure 26.4 A–D*. In the 6th week (*Figure 26.4A*), the mandibular dental lamina appears in front of the tongue primordium and above Meckel's cartilage. In the 7th week (*Figure 26.4B*), the vestibular lamina makes its appearance. One of the tooth buds formed by the dental lamina is shown. Here the ectoderm has attracted ectomesenchymal (neural crest) cells to its immediate neighborhood. By the 10th week (*Figure 26.4C*), the vestibular lamina has excavated the mesoderm, creating the vestibule. The tooth bud is in the 'cap' stage of development, the ectoderm being arranged like a

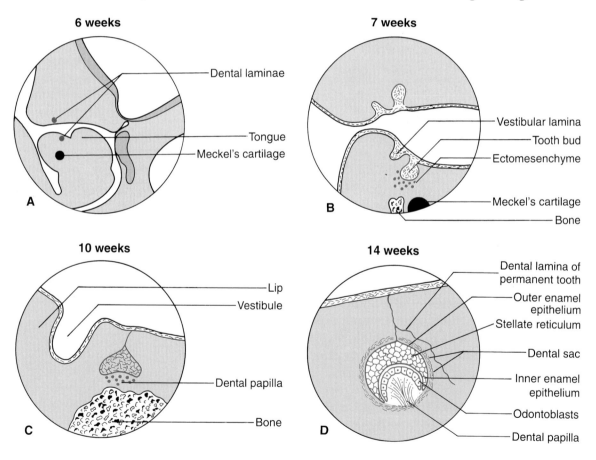

Figure 26.4. Early tooth development. (A) Dental lamina stage (see also *Figure 24.9A*). (B) Bud stage. (C) Cap stage. (D) Bell stage.

cap over a *dental papilla* formed by the ectomesoderm.

By the 14th week (*Figure 26.4D*), the tooth bud is in the 'bell' stage of development. The bell-shaped ectoderm is now an *enamel organ*, comprising an *outer* and an *inner enamel epithelium* separated by a *stellate reticulum*. The inner epithelium has induced the underlying mesenchyme to develop a layer of *odontoblasts*. A surrounding shell of mesenchyme has condensed as the *dental sac*. The dental sac and its contents constitute the *tooth germ*.

The cord of cells still linked to the surface ectoderm gives off dental laminae that will initiate the germs of the permanent teeth.

The germs of the permanent molars appear in postnatal life. They arise from dental laminae that burrow back into the posterior part of the jaws (*Figure 26.3C*).

Crowns (Figure 26.5A)

The odontoblasts form **predentin**, which later calcifies to become the **dentin** of the

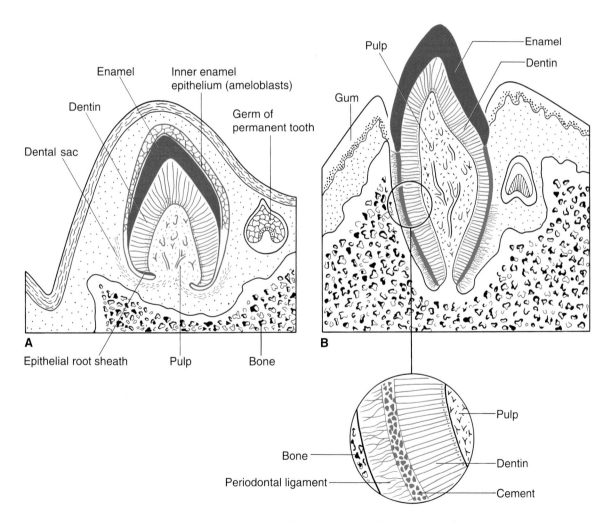

Figure 26.5. Mandibular deciduous incisor tooth. (A) Crown. (B) Crown and root.

tooth. (The spellings predentine and dentine are often used instead.) Calcification of the predentin is a signal for the cells of the inner enamel epithelium to become *ameloblasts*, which are responsible for laying down **enamel** on the surface of the dentin.

The central cells of the dental papilla constitute the **pulp** of the tooth, which is richly supplied with blood vessels and sensory nerve endings.

All of the structures formed thus far constitute the **crown** of the tooth.

Roots (Figure 26.5B)

Deep to the level of enamel production, the outer and inner enamel epithelia come together, as the *epithelial root sheath*. This sheath extends into the subjacent mesenchyme. Predentin and dentin are induced as before, to form the **root** of the tooth. (The number of roots to a tooth depends on whether one, two or three epithelial root sheaths are formed.) In the absence of any stellate reticulum within the sheath, ameloblasts are not formed by the inner epithelial layer of the root sheath. Instead, mesoderm of the dental sac produces a specialized form of bone, called **cement**. Outside the cement, the dental sac forms the **periodontal ligament**, which anchors the cement to the wall of the bony alveolus (socket) in which the tooth comes to lie.

Eruption

At birth, the crowns of the 20 deciduous teeth are partly calcified and the roots have yet to form. With postnatal growth of the roots, the crowns are progressively pushed toward the oral cavity. The enamel organs atrophy and their remnants are shed when the teeth erupt through the gums. Eruption normally spans the period between the 6th and 24th month after birth, commencing with the incisors and terminating with the second deciduous molars.

SALIVARY GLANDS

The **parotid gland** originates as a bud of ectodermal cells within the vestibule, near the corner of the stomodeum. The bud burrows into the maxillary mesenchyme, becoming a stem that gives off numerous branches in front of the ear. The stem becomes the hollow **parotid duct**, and the branches give rise to the **alveoli** of the gland during the middle trimester.

The **submandibular** and **sublingual** salivary glands develop in a manner similar to the parotid. They originate as outgrowths from oral endoderm under cover of the tongue (see *Figure 25.4*). The acini develop from the duct epithelium during the middle trimester.

MALFORMATIONS

Chondrocranium

In several inherited disorders, including Down's syndrome, cretinism and achondroplasia, growth activity at the spheno-occipital synchondrosis is deficient. In consequence, the middle region of the face fails to protrude in the normal manner, and the brain tends to overhang as shown by bulging frontal prominences (bossing).

Vault

The *size* of the vault is determined by the volume of the cranial contents. In *hydrocephaly*, which features ballooning of the ventricles of the brain (Chapter 29), the calvaria may become enormous in the absence of treatment; the individual bones continue to expand and the sutures remain separate. Conversely, in *microcephaly*, caused by underdevelopment of the brain (Chapter 30), the sutures and fontanelles unite prematurely.

The *shape* of the vault is influenced by the growth of the chondrocranium, to which it is attached around its margins. As already mentioned, a reduced chondrocranium is associated with abnormal 'bossing' of the frontal bones.

Premature fusion (*craniostenosis*) of certain calvarial sutures can lead to considerable distortion, because the continued growth of the brain becomes directed toward the sutures that remain open. For example, premature fusion of the sagittal suture results in a skull that is narrow from side to side and long anteroposteriorly. Premature union of the coronal suture causes an opposite effect: the skull becomes short anteroposteriorly and pointed on top.

Viscerocranium

Micrognathia is the condition in which the mandible is too small. It is observed in several inherited disorders and is attributed to faulty growth of neural crest cells contributing to the mandibular arch mesenchyme. The maxillae and zygomatic bones (also derived from the first arch) may be equally small.

Teeth

Abnormalities of the teeth often have a hereditary trait which affects the shape, number and position of the teeth; enamel and dentin formation may also show inherited defects.

EMBRYOLOGICAL TERMS

Otic capsule. Occipital sclerotomes. Parachordal cartilages. Hypophysial cartilages. Prechordal cartilages. Alisphenoid. Orbitosphenoid. Nasal capsule. Tooth buds. Enamel epithelium. Stellate reticulum. Dental sac. Tooth germ. *Microcephaly. Craniostenosis. Micrognathia.*

27

Head and neck: the ear

AURICLE

The auricle (pinna) develops from six *aural hillocks*, three of them located on the first pharyngeal arch and three on the second. They are depicted in *Figure 25.1*. The pinna is initially (6th week) located in the upper part of the neck. It is displaced cranially later on, during development of the ramus of the mandible.

EXTERNAL ACOUSTIC MEATUS *(Figure 27.1)*

From the first pharyngeal cleft, an ectodermal diverticulum, the **external acoustic meatus** (outer ear canal) extends inward toward the pharynx during the 5th week. Until the 18th week, the diverticulum contains a plug of ectodermal cells. The plug resolves into the stratified squamous lining of the canal and of the outer surface of the ear drum.

TYMPANIC CAVITY AND ITS CONTENTS *(Figure 27.1)*

The middle ear cavity develops from the blind end of the *tubotympanic recess*, which extends outward from the first pharyngeal pouch during the 5th week. The recess

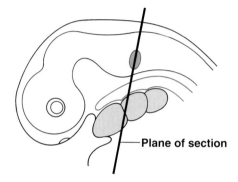

Plane of section

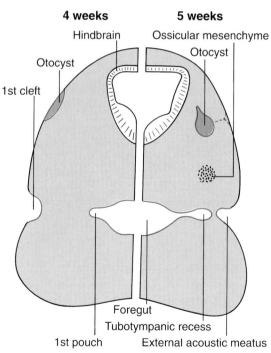

Figure 27.1. Early development of the ear.

makes contact with the outer ear canal, and the film of mesoderm between the two blind tubes is the primordium of the **tympanic membrane** (ear drum). The outer end of the tubotympanic recess expands to form the **tympanic cavity**. The stalk of the recess persists as the **pharyngotympanic tube** (Eustachian tube).

The **ossicles** develop from the dorsal ends of the first and second branchial arches. At first, the mesenchymal primordia lie above the tympanic cavity (*Figure 27.1*). The cavity gradually enlarges to incorporate them into the middle ear, conferring an epithelial lining on them as it does so (*Figure 27.2*).

The **tensor tympani** muscle differentiates from the first arch mesoderm, in company with the **malleus** and **incus**. The **stapedius** differentiates from the second arch, together with the **stapes**.

INNER EAR

At the end of the 3rd week, a patch of thickened ectoderm, the *otic placode*, appears beside the hindbrain. The otic placode sinks beneath the surface and forms the *otic vesicle* (*otocyst*) (*Figure 27.1*). A diverticulum sprouts from the otocyst, and becomes the **endolymphatic duct and sac** (*Figure 27.3A,B*). The otocyst itself becomes 8-shaped, showing a *vestibular sac* and a *cochlear sac* (*Figure 27.3B*). From the vestibular sac, three plate-like expansions give rise to the **semicircular ducts**; the remainder of the sac persists as the **utricle** (*Figure 27.3C*). The epithelial lining of the ducts and sac differentiates into the hair cells and ancillary structures of the three ampullary cristae and of the **utricular macula**.

From the cochlear sac arises the coiled **cochlear duct**. The remainder of this sac

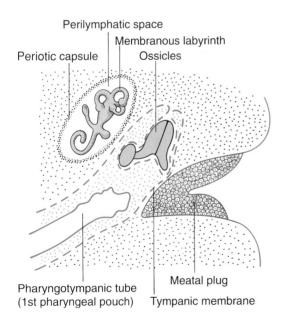

Figure 27.2. Later development of the ear. Dashed line indicates impending extension of the first pharyngeal pouch to surround the ossicles.

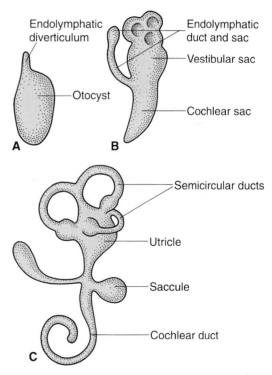

Figure 27.3. Development of the membranous labyrinth.

persists as the **saccule** (*Figure 27.3C*). The epithelial lining of the duct and sac differentiates into the hair cells and ancillary structures of the **organ of Corti** and of the **saccular macula**. The above transformations of the otic vesicle complete the **membranous labyrinth**, which is entirely ectodermal in origin, and contains **endolymph**.

The **bony labyrinth** results from the ossification of the *periotic capsule*, a shell of chondrified mesoderm surrounding the membranous labyrinth (*Figure 27.2*). Loose mesenchyme enclosed by the capsule breaks down to provide a space filled with **perilymph**.

VESTIBULOCOCHLEAR NERVE

Vestibular and cochlear nerve cells differentiate from the wall of the otocyst, which includes some cells from the neural crest. They are bipolar neurons.

The somas of the vestibular neurons finally occupy the outer end of the internal acoustic meatus. Their peripheral processes innervate the hair cells contained in the five sense organs of the membranous labyrinth. Their central processes enter the brain stem at the junction of pons and medulla oblongata, and synapse in the vestibular nucleus.

The somas of the cochlear neurons finally occupy the central pillar (modiolus) of the cochlea. Their peripheral processes innervate the hair cells of the spiral organ (of Corti). Their central processes travel alongside those of the vestibular division and synapse in the cochlear nucleus.

SUMMARY

The component parts of the ear, and their embryonic origins, are summarized in *Table 27.1*).

Table 27.1 Origins of the component parts of the ear

Component	Origin
Auricle	Pharyngeal arches 1 and 2
External acoustic meatus	1st pharyngeal cleft
Middle ear	Tubotympanic recess
Ossicles and muscles	1st pharyngeal arch (malleus, incus, tensor tympani) 2nd pharyngeal arch (stapes, stapedius)
Inner ear	Otocyst
VIII nerve	Otocyst, neural crest

The Ear at Birth

The inner ear, the tympanic cavity and the ossicles are almost fully adult in size at birth. So too is the **tympanic antrum**, an upward extension of the tympanic cavity. On the other hand, the mastoid process has not yet appeared.

The upper part of the tympanic membrane leans laterally at birth. The outer ear canal is relatively short, and care must be taken to avoid damage to the ear drum when approaching it with a speculum.

MALFORMATIONS

Congenital Deafness

All forms of deafness, whether congenital or acquired, fall into two categories. *Conductive deafness* is caused by disease of the outer or middle ear. *Sensorineural deafness* is caused by disease of the cochlea and/or of the central auditory pathways.

Congenital deafness resulting from maldevelopment of the *outer ear* is rare. It results from *meatal atresia*, where the ear canal is narrow and the meatal plate never becomes canalized. Meatal atresia may be part of a first arch syndrome associated with underdevelopment of mandibular arch elements.

Congenital deafness from middle ear malformations is also rare. Again, it may be part of a first arch syndrome associated with maldevelopment of the malleus and/or incus. *Congenital fixation of the stapes* may occur as an isolated phenomenon causing severe conductive deafness in one or both ears; the footplate of the stapes is firmly anchored in the oval window because of failure of the annular ligament to develop.

Congenital sensorineural deafness may be hereditary or acquired. *Hereditary deafness* is usually a recessive Mendelian trait when severe, and a dominant trait when it is mild.

The anatomical defects of the cochlea vary with different traits, and some are associated with abnormal pigmentation of the hair or of the irises. *Acquired deafness* is notoriously associated with exposure of the mother to the virus of rubella (German measles) during the second month of pregnancy. In the past, acquired deafness has also been caused by administration of streptomycin or thalidomide.

EMBRYOLOGICAL TERMS

Aural hillocks. Meatal plate. Tubotympanic recess. Otic placode. Otocyst. Vestibular sac. Cochlear sac. Periotic capsule. *Meatal atresia*. *Congenital fixation of the stapes*.

28

Head and neck: the eye

OPTIC VESICLE, LENS VESICLE

Two key events in ocular development take place early in the 4th week. First, the *optic vesicle* develops as an outgrowth of the diencephalon, the stem of the vesicle being the *optic stalk (Figure 28.1A)*. Secondly, under the inductive influence of the optic vesicle, the *lens vesicle* develops as an ingrowth of a thickened patch of surface ectoderm, the *lens placode*.

OPTIC CUP, OPTIC FISSURE

As the lens vesicle sinks inward, the optic vesicle becomes a double-walled *optic cup*, which receives the vesicle *(Figure 28.1B)*. Invagination of the optic cup extends along the under surface of the cup and stalk, creating the optic fissure *(Figure 28.2)*.

VITREOUS. CENTRAL VESSELS OF RETINA

The optic fissure is infiltrated by mesenchyme before its lips come together dur-ing the 6th week. Within the cup, the mesenchyme produces a gelatinous secretion that fills the **vitreous compartment of the eye** *(Figures 28.3* and *28.4)*. *Hyaloid vessels* also develop from the mesenchyme; they pass through the vitreous chamber and nourish the immature lens. As the lens matures, the distal parts of the hyaloid vessels atrophy, their course being represented permanently by the **hyaloid canal** crossing the vitreous. Their proximal parts form the **central vessels of the retina**. These two features are shown in *Figure 28.6*.

VASCULAR AND FIBROUS COATS. EXTRAOCULAR MUSCLES *(Figure 28.4)*

During the 5th and 6th weeks, the outer surface of the optic cup is invested with a shell of mesenchyme. Some of the mesenchyme is derived from prechordal mesoderm (Chapter 25); the remainder is ectomesenchyme derived from the rostral extremity of the neural crest. The mesenchymal shell differentiates into the vascular, **choroid coat** of the eyeball and the fibrous coat composed of the **sclera** and **cornea**. The **extraocular**

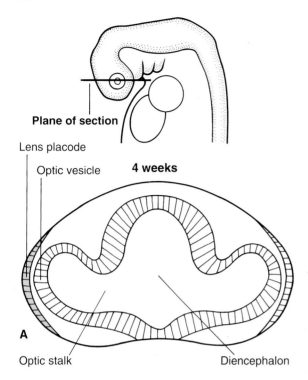

Plane of section

Lens placode

Optic vesicle   **4 weeks**

A

Optic stalk   Diencephalon

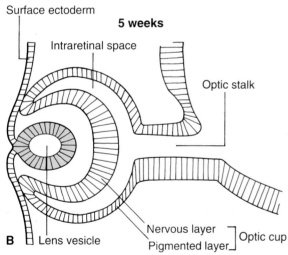

Surface ectoderm

5 weeks

Intraretinal space

Optic stalk

B Lens vesicle

Nervous layer ⎤ Optic cup
Pigmented layer ⎦

Figure 28.1. Early development of the eye.

muscles (the four rectus muscles and the two obliques) develop from loose, prechordal mesoderm outside the shell.

At the level of junction of sclera with cornea, the vascular coat forms the bulk of the **ciliary body**, including the **ciliary muscle** and **ciliary processes**. Anterior to the lens, it forms the connective tissue of the iris. The smooth muscles of the iris (**sphincter and dilator pupillae**) differentiate from the neurectoderm lining its posterior surface (see below).

LENS (*Figures 28.4 and 28.5*)

The cells in the posterior wall of the lens vesicle elongate and lay down *primary lens fibers*. Later, *secondary lens fibers* are laid down by cells that migrate into the interior of the lens from a mitotic zone around the lens margin.

FATE OF THE OPTIC CUP (*Figures 28.5 and 28.6*)

The outer epithelium of the optic cup accumulates melanin pigment and becomes the **pigmented layer** of the retina. Around the rim of the cup, the outer and inner layers form the posterior epithelium of the ciliary body and iris.

The intrinsic ocular muscles are of ectodermal origin. The **ciliary muscle** develops from ectomesenchymal cells in the ciliary body, whereas the **sphincter and dilator pupillae muscles** develop from the posterior epithelium of the iris.

Most of the inner epithelium of the optic cup becomes the **nervous layer** of the retina (*Figure 28.7*). It differentiates into **photosensory cells**, **bipolar neurons**, and **ganglionic neurons**, together with internuncial neurons and neuroglial cells. The ganglionic cells number 1–1.5 million, and their centrally directed processes (axons) form the **nerve fiber layer** of the retina as they converge upon the optic stalk.

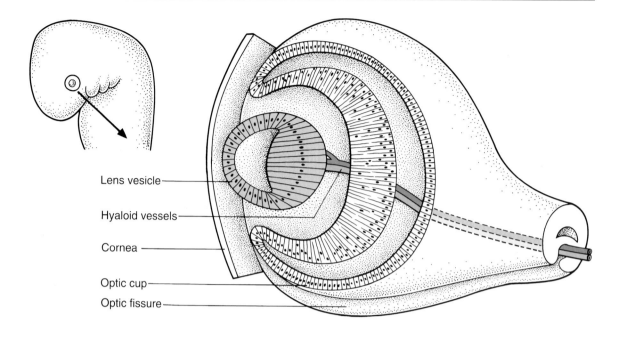

Figure 28.2. The eye at 6 weeks, showing the optic fissure.

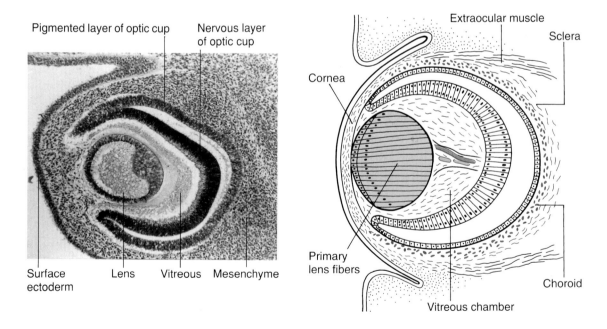

Figure 28.3. Sagittal section through the eye, at 6.5 weeks. (Cambridge Collection.)

Figure 28.4. The orbit at 8 weeks.

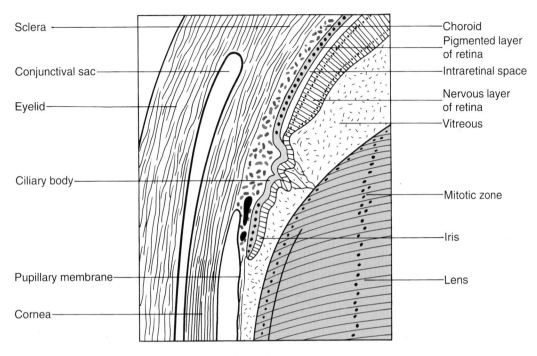

Figure 28.5. Later development of the anterior part of the eye.

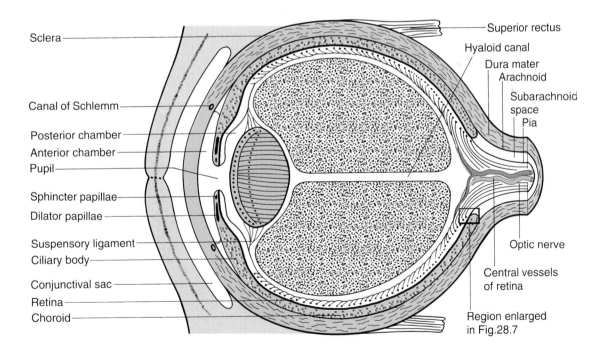

Figure 28.6. The eye at about 20 weeks.

OPTIC NERVE, CHIASM, TRACT

The optic fissure creates a direct conduit into the optic stalk, for the axons of the ganglionic cells. Without the fissure, there would be no escape from the optic cup save at its rim. The axons travel along the inner wall of the optic fissure as the **optic nerve**.

The two optic nerves come together in the ventral part of the lamina terminalis, as the **optic chiasm**. Axons from the nasal half of the retina cross the midline in the chiasm and join uncrossed axons originating in the opposite temporal half-retina. The crossed and uncrossed axons run together as the **optic tract**. About 90% of the tract fibers terminate in the **lateral geniculate nucleus** of the thalamus; the rest enter the midbrain where they have diverse terminations.

ANTERIOR AND POSTERIOR CHAMBERS (*Figures 28.5 and 28.6*)

The **aqueous humor** is secreted by the ciliary processes. It accumulates in the interval between the cornea and the lens. Initially, the vascular coat forms a *pupillary membrane* in front of the lens, but this disintegrates as the aqueous humor accumulates. It is then possible to identify the **anterior chamber** of the eye, located between iris and cornea, and the **posterior chamber**, between iris and lens. The aqueous humor moves from posterior to anterior chamber through the **pupil**. It passes from the anterior chamber into the **sinus venosus sclerae** (canal of Schlemm), a small vein encircling the eye at the anterior margin of the choroid coat.

MENINGEAL SHEATH OF THE OPTIC NERVE (*Figure 28.7*)

The optic nerve is not a true peripheral nerve. It is an extension of the white matter of the central nervous system. Like white matter elsewhere, it is invested with a meningeal sheath. The **leptomeninges** (pia mater, arachnoid mater) originate from neural crest cells. The **dura mater** is probably derived from prechordal mesoderm.

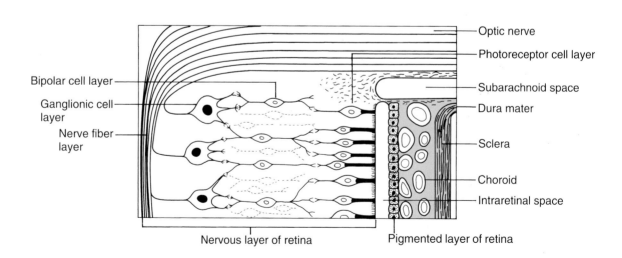

Bipolar cell layer

Ganglionic cell layer

Nerve fiber layer

Nervous layer of retina

Optic nerve

Photoreceptor cell layer

Subarachnoid space

Dura mater

Sclera

Choroid

Intraretinal space

Pigmented layer of retina

Figure 28.7. Schematic enlargement from the region of the box in *Figure 28.6*.

EYELIDS AND LACRIMAL APPARATUS

The **eyelids** are mesodermal folds, lined by surface ectoderm, that grow to meet each other in front of the cornea during the second month of gestation. From the 3rd to 6th months, the conjunctival sac is sealed by fusion of the apposed epithelial edges of the lids.

The **lacrimal gland** develops from the outer part of the conjunctival sac, in the manner of exocrine glands elsewhere. Although a crying infant is not tearful, a continuous lacrimal secretion is present in order to protect the cornea.

SUMMARY OF ECTODERMAL CONTRIBUTIONS TO THE ORBIT

Surface ectoderm forms the lens; the stratified squamous epithelium lining the conjunctival sac and the outer surface of the cornea; the secretory cells and ducts of the lacrimal gland, and of the tarsal glands (within the eyelids); and the hair follicles that produce the eyelashes. *Neurectoderm* forms the optic cup and its derivatives: retina; epithelial lining of ciliary body and posterior surface of iris; sphincter and dilator pupillae. (The epithelium governing the secretion of aqueous humor is derived from the nervous layer of the optic cup.) The earliest cells of the vitreous are shed from the nervous layer of the cup; later cells come from the mesoderm surrounding the hyaloid vessels. *Neural crest ectomesenchyme* forms the pigmented cells in the stroma of the uveal tract (choroid, ciliary body, iris); also the ciliary muscle, and the leptomeningeal investment of the optic nerve. The extent of the neural crest contribution to the connective tissue of the sclera and cornea is uncertain.

MALFORMATIONS

In *anophthalmia*, the eyeball is absent or only rudimentary on one or both sides. The condition is the result of more or less complete failure of development of the optic vesicle. *Cyclopia* is a very rare condition where the optic outgrowths fuse within a single, median orbit; concomitant malformations of the brain are incompatible with life.

Coloboma of the iris is a condition resulting from incomplete closure of the optic fissure during the 7th week of development. Minor degrees of coloboma are fairly common, the pupil having the shape of a keyhole. Major degrees are associated with wedge-shaped defects in the iris, ciliary body, retina and even the optic nerve.

Partial *persistence of the pupillary membrane* is not uncommon. Vision is usually not affected.

Congenital cataract (opacity of the lens, with blindness) is the result of abnormal development of lens fibers, notably during the 7th week of development. The abnormality may be genetic in origin, or may be brought about by a teratogenic agent – notably, the virus of rubella (German measles).

Persistence of hyaloid vessels is often noted on clinical examination of the posterior chamber of the eye. Rarely, embryonic connective tissue persists around the vessels, with severe obstruction of vision.

EMBRYOLOGICAL TERMS

Optic vesicle, optic stalk. Lens placode, lens vesicle. Optic cup, optic fissure. Hyaloid vessels. Primary and secondary lens fibers. *Anophthalmia. Cyclopia. Coloboma. Persistent pupillary membrane. Congenital cataract. Persistent hyaloid vessels.*

29

Head and neck: general features of brain development

BRAIN VESICLES

Before the end of the 4th week of development (Chapter 8), the rostral part of the neural tube shows three expansions known as *primary brain vesicles*: the *prosencephalon* (**forebrain**), the *mesencephalon* (**midbrain**), and the *rhombencephalon* (**hindbrain**) (*Figure 29.1A*).

The brain stem buckles as development proceeds. A *cervical flexure* appears at the junction of the brain stem and spinal cord, and a *midbrain flexure* moves the mesencephalon to the summit of the brain (*Figure 29.1B*). A little later, the rhombencephalon folds upon itself at the *pontine flexure*, causing the walls of the neural tube to flare, thus creating the **fourth ventricle** of the brain (*Figure 29.1C*). The rhomboid (diamond) shape of the fourth ventricle gives the rhombencephalon its name.

The dorsal region of the prosencephalon expands on each side to form the *telencephalon* (**cerebral hemispheres**). The remainder, straddling the midline, is the *diencephalon* (*Figures 29.1C* and *29.2*). The *optic outgrowth* from the diencephalon is the forerunner of the retina and optic nerve (Chapter 28).

The diencephalon, mesencephalon and rhombencephalon constitute the embryonic brain stem.

The rostral part of the rhombencephalon gives rise to the **pons** and **cerebellum**. The caudal part gives rise to the **medulla oblongata**.

VENTRICULAR SYSTEM (*Figures 29.3 and 29.4*)

The neural canal dilates within the cerebral hemispheres, forming the **lateral ventricles**. The **third ventricle** is the cavity within the diencephalon, bounded rostrally by the thin **lamina terminalis** which represents the site of closure of the rostral neuropore. Each lateral ventricle communicates with the third ventricle through an **interventricular foramen**. The third and fourth ventricles communicate through the **aqueduct** of the midbrain.

Choroid Plexuses

The thin roof plates of the forebrain and hindbrain are invaginated by tufts of capil-

3.5 weeks

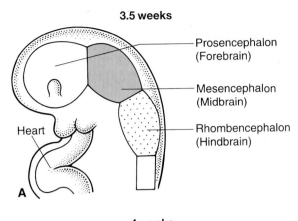

Prosencephalon
(Forebrain)

Mesencephalon
(Midbrain)

Rhombencephalon
(Hindbrain)

Heart

A

4 weeks

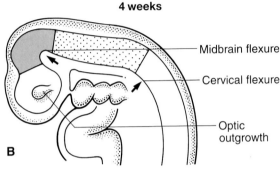

Midbrain flexure

Cervical flexure

Optic
outgrowth

B

6 weeks

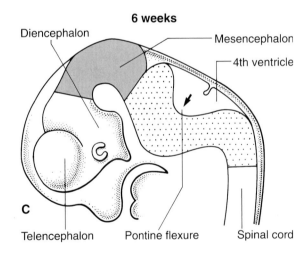

Diencephalon

Mesencephalon

4th ventricle

Telencephalon   Pontine flexure   Spinal cord

C

Figure 29.1. Early development of the brain.

laries which form the **choroid plexuses** (*Figure 29.3*). A filtrate of the choroid plexuses provides **cerebrospinal fluid** which flows through the ventricular system. The fluid escapes through one **median aper-**

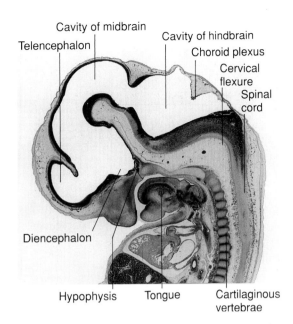

Cavity of midbrain
Telencephalon

Cavity of hindbrain
Choroid plexus
Cervical flexure
Spinal cord

Diencephalon

Hypophysis   Tongue   Cartilaginous vertebrae

Figure 29.2. Median section of head and thorax, at 6 weeks. (Carnegie Collection.)

ture and two **lateral apertures** in the roof plate of the fourth ventricle, to enter the subarachnoid space.

BRAIN STEM

In the embryonic midbrain, pons and medulla oblongata the walls of the neural tube have much in common with the embryonic spinal cord (*Figure 29.4*). Basal and alar plates can be identified, each of them exhibiting ventricular, intermediate and marginal zones. In the mesencephalon, the central canal is enclosed by the plates, which in due course form the **periaqueductal gray matter**. In the rhombencephalon, on the other hand, the ventricular zone contributes only ependymal cells to the stretched-out roof plate, and the central gray matter occupies the floor of the fourth ventricle.

Choroidal vessels develop in the pia mater overlying the ventricular roof plate. As they

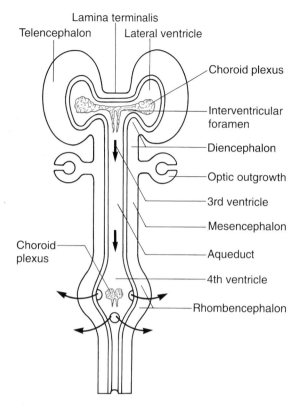

Lamina terminalis

Telencephalon   Lateral ventricle

Choroid plexus

Interventricular foramen

Diencephalon

Optic outgrowth

3rd ventricle

Mesencephalon

Choroid plexus

Aqueduct

4th ventricle

Rhombencephalon

Figure 29.3. Ventricular system of the brain. Arrows indicate flow of cerebrospinal fluid secreted by the choroid plexuses.

invaginate through the roof, they receive an ependymal coat which becomes the **choroidal epithelium** covering the choroid plexus within the ventricle.

The neuroblasts of the basal plate form the motor nuclei of cranial nerves. Those of the alar plate form the sensory nuclei of cranial nerves, and the **superior and inferior colliculi** of the midbrain. In the upper part of the rhombencephalon, the dorsal lip of the alar plate becomes swollen with neuroblasts destined to form the cerebellum (see below).

Cells also migrate from the alar plate into the area ventral to the central gray matter, known as the **tegmentum**; here they form the **red nucleus** of the midbrain, the **nuclei pontis** in the pons, and the **olive** in the

medulla oblongata. Other alar-plate neuroblasts mature into the **aminergic neurons** of the **substantia nigra**, **raphe nuclei**, and **locus ceruleus**. The aminergic neurons form terminal varicosities within their target territories, including the cerebral hemispheres, before the end of the embryonic period, and they are believed to provide *growth factors* necessary for maturation of the brain.

Details of cranial nerve development are in Chapter 30.

CEREBELLUM

In the rostral part of the rhombencephalon, the margins of the flared alar plates curl inward to form a *rhombic lip* on each side (*Figure 29.4*). Neuroblasts in the rhombic lips proliferate and meet in the midline to complete the *cerebellar primordium*.

Initial enlargement of the cerebellum takes place within the fourth ventricle (*Figure 29.5*). The so-called 'eversion' of the cerebellar rudiment is the result of the later rapid growth of the extraventricular portion. Lateral expansions form the **cerebellar hemispheres**; the part remaining in the midline region forms the **vermis** (*Figures 29.6* and *29.7*).

Histogenesis of the cerebellar gray matter is described in the next chapter.

FOREBRAIN

General Features

Developing neurons migrate from the ventricular zone of the telencephalon to the surface, where they form the **cerebral cortex**. (For details, see next chapter.)

Expansion of the cerebral hemispheres is not uniform. A region on the lateral surface on each side, the **insula** (*Figure 29.8*), is rela-

tively quiescent and forms a pivot around which the expanding hemisphere rotates. **Frontal**, **parietal**, **occipital** and **temporal lobes** can be identified at 12–14 weeks.

A C-shaped arrangement of certain structures is brought about by the downward and forward extension of the temporal lobe. On the medial surface of the hemisphere, a patch of cerebral cortex, the **hippocampus**, is separated from the roof plate of the third ventricle by the developing choroid plexus of the forebrain (*Figure 29.9A*). Most of the hippocampus is drawn into the temporal lobe, leaving in its wake a strand of nerve fibers called the **fornix**. Next to the fornix is the **choroid fissure**, through which the

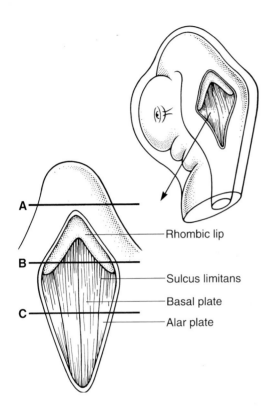

Rhombic lip

Sulcus limitans

Basal plate

Alar plate

Figure 29.4. Early and late phases of brain stem development. Paired arrows in (B) indicate migration of the cerebellar primordia into the roof of the fourth ventricle. CC, crus cerebri; CGM, central gray matter; CNN, cranial nerve nuclei; ION, inferior olivary nucleus; NP, nuclei pontis; PAG, periaqueductal gray matter; RN, red nucleus; SC, superior colliculus; SN, substantia nigra.

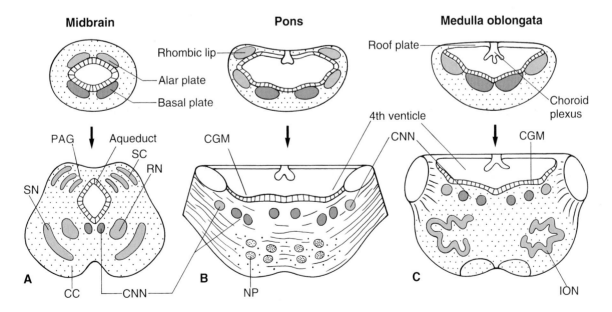

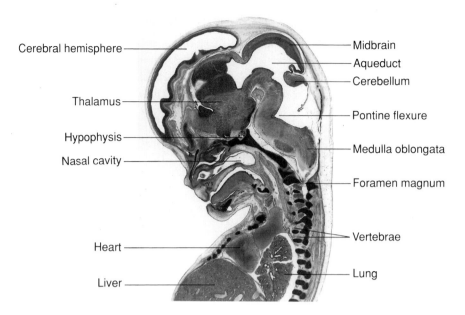

Figure 29.5. Median section through head and thorax, at 10 weeks. (Carnegie Collection.)

choroid plexus invaginates into the lateral ventricle. Also shown is the caudate nucleus, which becomes comma-shaped when its tail is drawn into the temporal lobe (*Figure 29.9B*).

The **anterior commissure** develops as a connection linking olfactory (smell) regions of the left and right sides. Above this, a much larger commissure, the **corpus callosum** links matching areas of the cerebral cortex of the two sides. It extends backward above the fornix. A remnant of hippocampal gray matter remains as the **induseum griseum** on the upper surface of the corpus callosum. The medial wall of both hemispheres is thinned out in the interval between corpus callosum and fornix, to become the **septum pellucidum**.

Choroid Plexuses

The roof plate of the diencephalon consists of ependymal cells, covered by a film of pia mater in which the choroid plexus is embed-

ded (*Figure 29.10A*). The choroid plexus invaginates first through the roof and then laterally, to form the choroid plexuses of the third and lateral ventricles. As with the fourth ventricle, the ependymal coating of the choroidal capillaries becomes the specialized, choroidal epithelium which governs the composition of the cerebrospinal fluid.

A new roof for the third ventricle is provided by the fornix and corpus callosum (*Figure 29.10C*). The under surfaces of these two are lined by pia mater, with the result that vessels developing in this region (including the great cerebral vein) are covered above as well as below by pia mater. The double layer of pia is known as the **velum interpositum**.

Diencephalon

The diencephalon occupies the lateral wall of the third ventricle. It comprises **epithala-**

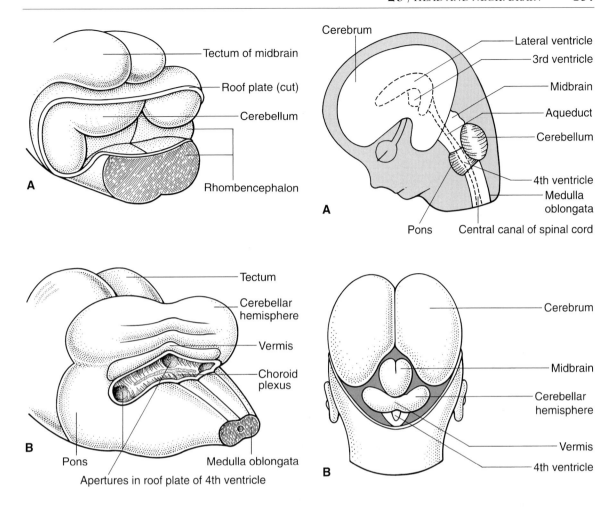

Figure 29.6. Hindbrain. (A) At 8 weeks, with roof plate of fourth ventricle removed. (B) At 12 weeks, with roof plate in place.

Figure 29.7 The brain at 12 weeks. (A) Side view. (B) Posterior view.

mus, thalamus, and **hypothalamus** (*Figure 29.10*). The epithalamus remains small, giving rise to the **pineal gland**, and the **posterior and habenular commissures**. The thalamus is made up of a large number (about 30) of separate nuclei. Some have general sensory functions (notably the ventral posterior); some have special sense functions (the medial geniculate serves hearing and the lateral geniculate serves vision); and some are involved in movement control (notably the ventral lateral). The hypothala-

mus is made up of some 20 separate nuclei serving functions primarily related to survival of the individual and of the species. Many of these functions are implemented through control of the pituitary gland (see next chapter).

Basal Ganglia

The term 'basal ganglia' was originally used to describe all of the nuclear masses located

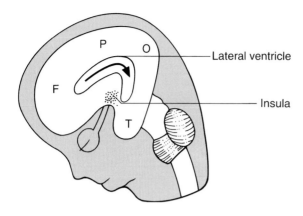

Figure 29.8. Arrow in lateral ventricle indicates C-shaped growth of the cerebral hemisphere around the insula. F, P, O, T, frontal, parietal, occipital, temporal lobes. (The occipital lobe, and the occipital horn of the lateral ventricle, are the last to form.)

in the basal region of the cerebral hemisphere. The term is currently used to designate four nuclei – one of them in the midbrain – concerned with the control of movement. These are the **striatum**, the **pallidum**, the **subthalamic nucleus** (which develops directly below the thalamus), and the **substantia nigra**.

In *Figure 29.11A*, the striatum is seen in the floor of the lateral ventricle. This nuclear mass develops from the ventricular zone and it enlarges *in situ*. It is incompletely divided by axons that grow from the thalamus into the cerebral cortex, forming the **internal capsule** and **corona radiata** (*Figure 29.11B*). The term 'striatum' derives from the strands of gray matter that continue to link its two parts, the **caudate nucleus** and the

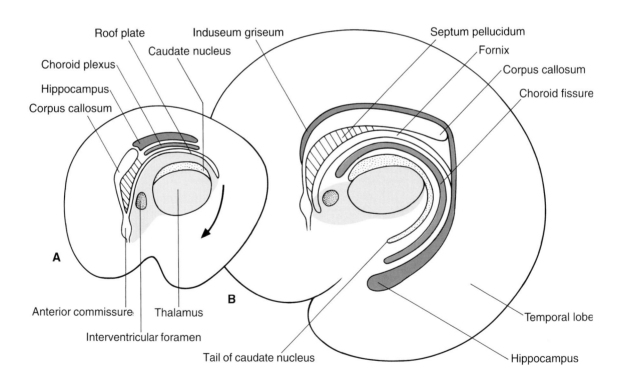

Figure 29.9. Diagram of the medial surface of the right hemisphere, illustrating the C-shaped arrangement of structures produced by forward extension of the temporal lobe.

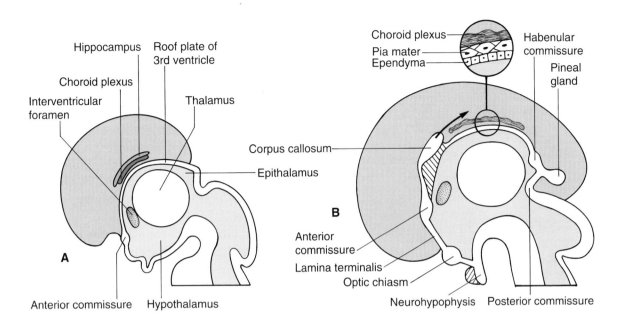

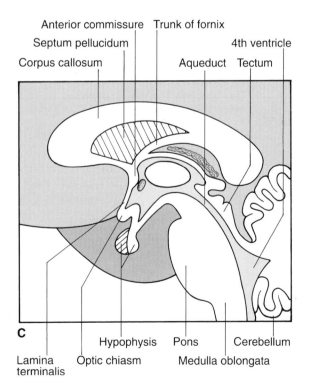

Figure 29.10. Median sections of the brain. (A) At 8 weeks. (B) At 12 weeks. (C) Postnatal.

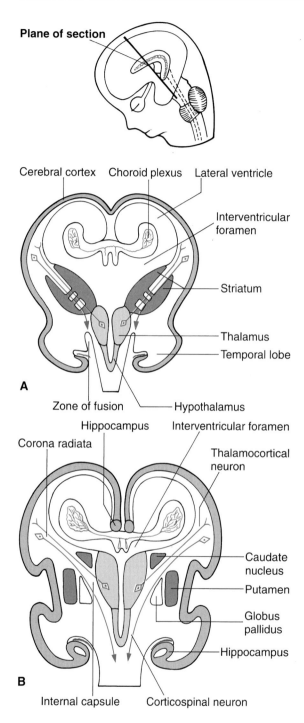

Figure 29.11. Coronal sections of the developing forebrain.

putamen. The caudate and putamen have the same microscopic structure, with a mixture of excitatory and inhibitory neurons.

The globus pallidus originates in the intermediate zone of the diencephalon. It becomes separated from the diencephalon by the internal capsule. A strand of pallidal cells becomes embedded in the cerebral peduncle, forming the *entopeduncular nucleus* in lower mammals, and the **substantia nigra**, **pars reticulata** in primates. In this context, the pigmented, dopaminergic neurons derived from the alar lamina of the midbrain constitute the **substantia nigra, pars compacta**. All of the pallidal neurons are inhibitory in nature.

Redefining the Brain Stem

The medial wall of the temporal lobe of the brain merges with the lateral wall of the diencephalon ('zone of fusion' in *Figure 29.11A*). In this way, the diencephalon is built into the cerebral hemisphere. One consequence is that the term 'brain stem' is restricted thereafter to the remaining, free parts of the embryonic brain stem: midbrain, pons and medulla oblongata. A second consequence is a broadening of the base of the brain allowing the cerebral cortex to project fibers direct to the brain stem. The most important of these projections is the **corticospinal tract**, which develops relatively late and is still unmyelinated at birth.

Sulci and Gyri

By the 28th week of development, several **sulci** (fissures) have appeared on the surface of the brain, notably the **lateral**, **central**, and **calcarine sulci** (*Figure 29.12*). All of the major sulci and **gyri** are present at birth.

Note: Malformations of the brain are described in the next chapter.

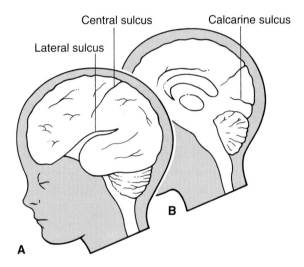

Figure 29.12. Three major sulci in the hemisphere of a 28-week fetus. (A) Lateral surface. (B) Medial surface.

EMBRYOLOGICAL TERMS

Prosencephalon. Mesencephalon. Rhombencephalon. Telencephalon. Diencephalon. Optic outgrowth. Cervical, midbrain, pontine flexures. Rhombic lip. Cerebellar primordium.

30

Head and neck: particular features of brain development

CRANIAL NERVES

Figure 30.1 illustrates the state of development of the cranial nerves at the end of the 6th week. The chief distributions of these nerves are summarized in *Table 30.1*.

Cell Columns

In the thoracic region of the developing spinal cord (Chapter 10), four distinct cell columns can be identified on each side. In the basal plate, the cell columns are *somatic efferent*, for the supply of the striated muscles of the trunk and limbs, and *general visceral efferent*, for the autonomic supply of the cardiovascular system. In the alar plate, a *general visceral afferent* column receives information from thoracic and abdominal organs, and a *somatic afferent* column receives information from the body wall.

In the brain stem, basal and alar plates can be identified, together with four cell columns corresponding to those of the cord. Three further columns occupy the brain stem (*Figure 30.2*):

- A *branchial (special visceral) efferent* column supplies striated muscle developing from the pharyngeal arches.
- A *special visceral afferent* column receives afferents from taste buds.
- A *special sense afferent* column receives afferents from the inner ear.

All seven columns provide efferent/afferent connections for one or more cranial nerves. Fragmentation of the columns is such that, in descriptions of individual cranial nerves, they are referred to as *nuclei*.

Cell Columns of the Basal Plate

SOMATIC EFFERENT CELL COLUMN
The somatic efferent nuclei are those of the **oculomotor**, **trochlear**, and **abducent nerves** for the extraocular muscles, and the **nucleus of the hypoglossal nerve** for the muscles of the tongue. All four occupy the central gray matter close to the midline.

BRANCHIAL EFFERENT CELL COLUMN
The cranial nerve nuclei concerned are the **motor nucleus of the trigeminal nerve** for

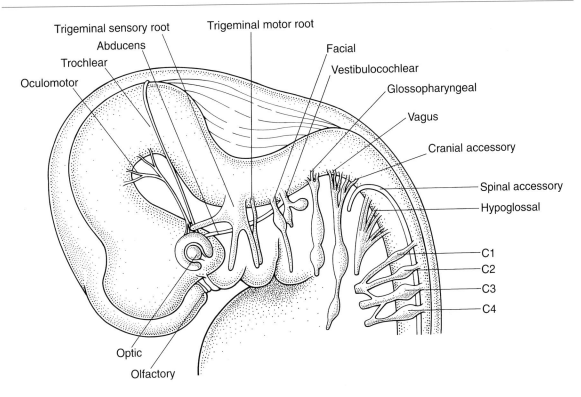

Figure 30.1. Cranial and upper cervical nerves at 6 weeks.

the muscles of mastication; the **main nucleus of the facial nerve** for the muscles of facial expression; and the **nucleus ambiguus** for the intrinsic muscles of the larynx and the pharyngeal constrictors. Axons emerge from the nucleus ambiguus in the **glossopharyngeal**, **vagus** and **cranial accessory nerves**. The nucleus itself migrates laterally, coming close to the spinal sensory nucleus of the trigeminal nerve (its main source of sensory stimulation).

A separate, hypobranchial muscle sheet gives rise to the sternomastoid and trapezius muscles. These are supplied by the **spinal accessory nucleus** which occupies the lateral part of the ventral gray matter in the five most cranial segments of the spinal cord.

General visceral efferent cell column
The outermost nuclear group in the basal plate corresponds to the intermediolateral

cell column of the spinal cord. It gives rise to the parasympathetic elements of certain cranial nerves: the **Edinger–Westphal nucleus**, the **superior and inferior salivatory nuclei**, the **cardioinhibitory nucleus** embedded in the rostral end of the nucleus ambiguus, and the **dorsal motor nucleus of the vagus**.

Cell Columns of the Alar Plate

General visceral afferent cell column
This cell column is represented by the lower part of the **nucleus solitarius**, which receives reflex afferents from the alimentary, respiratory and cardiovascular systems via the glossopharyngeal and vagus nerves.

Special visceral afferent cell column
This cell column is represented by the upper part of the **nucleus solitarius**, which

Nerves	Components		
	Sensory	Motor	Parasympathetic
I Olfactory	Olfactory epithelium		
II Optic	Retina		
III Oculomotor		Superior, medial, inferior rectus, inferior oblique	Sphincter of pupil, ciliary muscle (via ciliary ganglion)
IV Trochlear		Superior oblique	
V Trigeminal	Skin and mucous membranes of head	Muscles of mastication	
VI Abducens	Lateral rectus		
VII Facial	Palate and anterior tongue (taste)	Muscles of facial expression	Lacrimal gland (via pterygopalatine ganglion) Submandibular, sublingual glands (via submandibular ganglion)
VIII Vestibulocochlear	Sense organs of balance and hearing		
IX Glossopharyngeal	Oropharynx. Posterior tongue (taste). Carotid sinus, carotid body	Stylopharyngeus	Parotid gland (via otic ganglion)
X Vagus	Laryngopharynx, thoracic and abdominal viscera	Distributes fibers of cranial XI	Thoracic and abdominal organs (via intramural ganglia)
XI Accessory cranial		Muscles of larynx and pharynx	
spinal		Sternomastoid and trapezius	
XII hypoglossal		Muscles of tongue	

Table 30.1 Summary of cranial nerve distribution

receives gustatory afferents from the taste buds of the tongue and palate via the glossopharyngeal nerve.

SOMATIC AFFERENT CELL COLUMN

The **nuclei of the trigeminal nerve** receive somatic afferent information from the oronasal skin and mucous membranes and from the muscles of mastication, via the trigeminal nerve. (The so-called spinal nucleus of the trigeminal nerve, extending from lower pons to the third cervical segment of the spinal cord, receives nociceptive (pain) information, not only from trigeminal

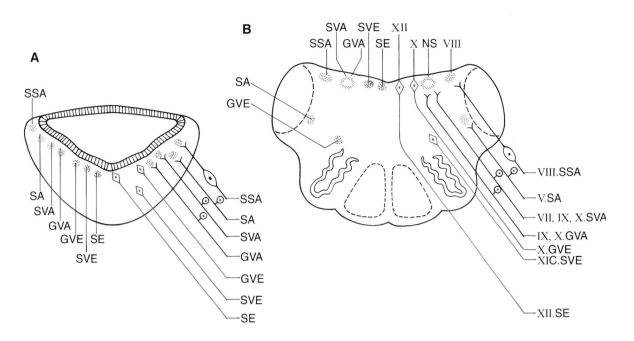

Figure 30.2. (A) Nerve cell columns in the embryonic hindbrain. (B) Counterparts in the adult medulla oblongata. *Cell columns*: SE, somatic efferent; SVE, special visceral efferent; GVE, general visceral efferent; GVA, general visceral afferent; SVA, special visceral afferent; SA, somatic afferent; SSA, special sense afferent. *Other labels*: NA, nucleus ambiguus; NS, nucleus solitarius; XIc, cranial XI nerve. *Note on n. solitarius*: The rostral part receives all afferents serving taste; the caudal part receives visceral afferents from the alimentary tract and respiratory tract.

territory, but also from the sensory territories of the glossopharyngeal, vagus and upper three spinal nerves.)

SPECIAL SENSE AFFERENT CELL COLUMN

This cell column is the most lateral of all. It is represented by the **vestibular nucleus** and by the **cochlear nucleus**, serving the special senses of balance and hearing, respectively. The special sense afferents concerned are bipolar neurons with cell bodies in the vestibular and cochlear ganglia.

Origin of Cranial Nerve Ganglia

The four cranial parasympathetic ganglia – ciliary, pterygopalatine, submandibular and otic – are derived from neural crest cells that migrate along the preganglionic fibers of the nerves concerned. The sensory ganglia attached to certain cranial nerves are derived in part from neural crest cells and in part from *placodes*. The placodes are localized thickenings of the surface ectoderm in the head region. Best known are the olfactory placode, which produces the bipolar neurons of the olfactory epithelium, the lens placode, which forms the lens of the eye, and the otic placode, which forms the membranous labyrinth of the inner ear and the bipolar neurons of the eighth cranial nerve. In addition, the *epibranchial placodes* (Chapter 24) contribute unipolar neurons to the sensory ganglia attached to the trigeminal, facial, glossopharyngeal and vagus nerves.

CEREBELLUM

Lobes

The first part of the cerebellum to appear is the **archicerebellum**, comprising the **nodule** in the midline and the **flocculus** on each side (*Figure 30.3*). Its central (efferent) nucleus is the fastigial. The cortex of this **flocculonodular** lobe has some direct, two-way connections with the nuclei of the vestibular nerves, reflecting its ancestral development (in fishes) in relation to the vestibular labyrinth.

The *paleocerebellum* appears next. This part is mainly confined to the **anterior lobe**; its central nuclei are the emboliform and globose, and its connections are chiefly spinal.

Phylogenetically the most recent, and the last and largest to appear, is the *neocerebellum*. This component forms the bulk of the **posterior lobe**. Its central nucleus is the dentate, and its connections are mainly with the cerebral cortex.

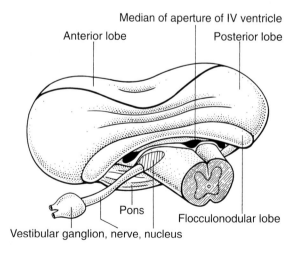

Median of aperture of IV ventricle
Anterior lobe   Posterior lobe

Pons
Flocculonodular lobe
Vestibular ganglion, nerve, nucleus

Figure 30.3. Posterior view of the rhombencephalon at 20 weeks.

Histodifferentiation

As was observed in Chapter 29, the cerebellum develops from the dorsal edge (rhombic lip) of the alar plate in the upper region of the rhombencephalon. From the rhombic lip, an *internal germinal layer* migrates along the ventricular surface of the cerebellar rudiment, and an *external germinal layer* migrates along the outer surface (*Figure 30.4A*). The internal layer gives rise to an intermediate zone (*Figure 30.4B*) which forms the **central nuclei** of the white matter (fastigial, emboliform, globose, dentate); also the **Purkinje cells** and **Golgi cells** of the cerebellar cortex (*Figure 30.4C,D*).

The external germinal layer engages in mitotic activity for a considerable period, and differentiates slowly. During the 6th month of gestation, this layer gives rise to **stellate** and **basket cells**, which mingle with the dendritic trees of Purkinje cells in the outer, **molecular layer** of the cortex. A little later, granule cells begin to migrate inward from it; the granule cells pass through the **piriform layer** of Purkinje cells and form the inner, **granular layer** of the cortex. The final number of granule cells has been reckoned at 30–50 billion, and the last ones are being formed as late as 6 months after birth. (The only other neurons showing any postnatal mitosis are the granule cells of the dentate gyrus in the temporal lobe of the cerebral hemisphere.)

HYPOPHYSIS

The hypophysis (pituitary gland) is entirely ectodermal in origin. The **adenohypophysis** (anterior lobe) arises from the roof of the stomodeum. The **neurohypophysis** (posterior lobe) arises from the floor of the diencephalon.

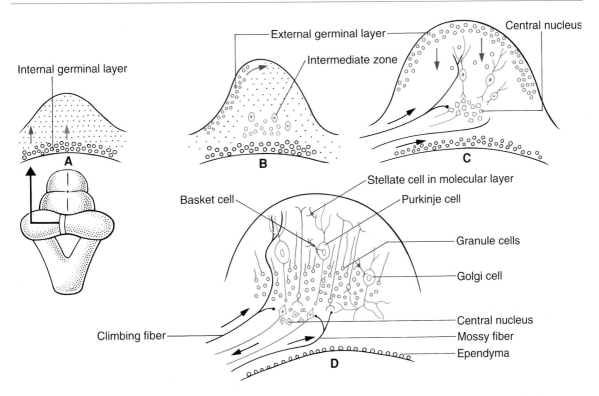

Figure 30.4. Histogenesis of the cerebellum. Red/blue arrows indicate cell migrations. Black arrows indicate nerve impulse conduction.

At the beginning of the 4th week, a hollow diverticulum known as *Rathke's pouch* ascends from the roof of the stomodeum into the mesenchyme beneath the brain (*Figure 30.5A*). At the same time, the **infundibulum** ('funnel') grows down from the diencephalon and is embraced by lateral expansions of Rathke's pouch.

The stalk of Rathke's pouch normally disappears. The anterior wall of the pouch enlarges, to become the **anterior lobe (adenohypophysis)** (*Figure 30.5B, C*). The cavity of the pouch persists as a narrow **cleft**. The posterior wall persists as the small, **middle lobe**. The **posterior lobe (neurohypophysis)** is formed by expansion of the lower end of the infundibulum (*Figure 30.6*).

The adenohypophysis develops into a typical endocrine gland comprising cell cords and a rich capillary bed. The main mass of cells forms the **pars distalis**, and the part embracing the neurohypophyseal downgrowth persists around the pituitary stalk as the **pars tuberalis** (*Figure 30.5D*). A portal system of vessels links the infundibular stalk to the pars distalis. **Parvocellular neuroendocrine cells** of the hypothalamus control the adenohypophyseal cells from the 20th week onward, by liberating releasing and inhibiting hormones into the portal system.

The neurohypophysis consists initially of neuroglial cells called **pituicytes**. However, **magnocellular neuroendocrine cells** of the hypothalamus send axons into the neurohypophysis (*Figure 30.5D*), and hormones are released into the capillary bed there from the 20th week onward.

Endocrine cells derived from the stalk of Rathke's pouch often persist in the mucous membrane lining the roof of the

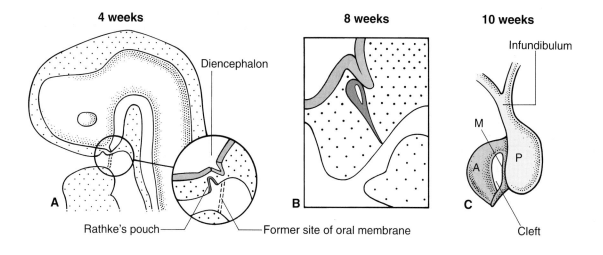

4 weeks

Diencephalon

Rathke's pouch ⎯⎯⎯⎯ Former site of oral membrane

A

8 weeks

B

10 weeks

Infundibulum

M

A   P

C

Cleft

20 weeks

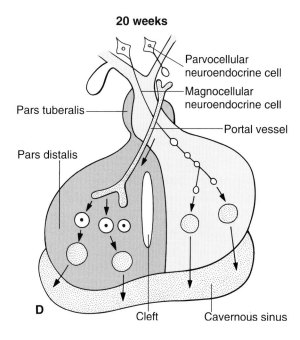

Parvocellular
neuroendocrine cell

Magnocellular
neuroendocrine cell

Pars tuberalis

Portal vessel

Pars distalis

D

Cleft   Cavernous sinus

Figure 30.5. Development of the hypophysis. A, anterior lobe; M, middle lobe; P, posterior lobe. Arrows indicate hormonal movements.

nasopharynx, as a small *pharyngeal hypophysis*. A *Rathke's pouch tumor*, or *craniopharyngioma*, is a well recognized tumor of childhood developing within or above the sphenoid bone.

TELENCEPHALON

The **cerebral cortex** develops by the migration of neuroblasts from the inner, ventricular zone of the telencephalon to the surface of the hemispheres, where they form a *cortical plate*. The migration occurs along radially disposed neuroglial-cell strands (*Figure 30.7*). The earliest parts of the cortex to appear are the oldest phylogenetically and include the **archicortex** of the pyriform lobe and the **allocortex** of the hippocampus. In these areas the cortex is three-layered. The remaining cortex – more than 90% of the whole – is the **neocortex**. The neocortex consists of six laminae. Lamina I is almost devoid of nerve cell bodies, which are abundant in laminae II–VI. A remarkable feature of neocortical development is its 'inside-out' nature. The first wave of young nerve cells to migrate along the radial fiber system are those destined for lamina VI. The second wave passes between the cells of lamina VI and forms lamina V. Further waves give rise to laminae IV, III and II in succession.

With the completion of cell division in the ventricular zone, the cells remaining there become **ependymal cells**. With the comple-

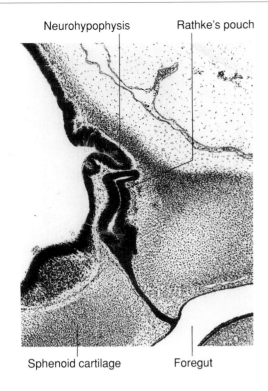

Figure 30.6. Hypophysis, at 6 weeks. (Taken from *Figure 29.2*.)

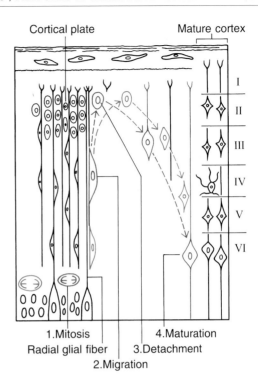

Figure 30.7. Scheme showing the inside-out pattern of development of the cerebral cortex. The horizontal cells in layer I disappear after birth.

tion of neuronal migration into the cortical plate, the radial glial fibers are lost and the parent cells become neuroglia. Following their arrival into their appropriate laminae, the young neurons emit axons and dendrites and make synaptic contacts. Some functional synaptic contacts are already present as early as the 7th week of development, at which time the embryo is capable of simple movements in response to external stimuli. Once maturation gets under way, cortical neurons are no longer capable of mitotic activity; the thickening of the cortex that takes place in the postnatal years is produced by proliferation of dendritic trees and branching of axons. Neuroglial cells continue to multiply well into the postnatal period. In later life they are the chief source of brain tumors.

BLOOD SUPPLY OF THE BRAIN

Arteries

The arterial blood supply to the brain develops from the cranial segments of the dorsal aortae, which constitute the two **internal carotid arteries**; also from the two **vertebral arteries**.

The arrangement of the major arteries at the end of the embryonic period is shown in *Figure 30.8A*. Upon reaching the brain, the internal carotid arteries turn dorsally and run alongside the diencephalon. They give off **anterior**, **middle** and **posterior cerebral arteries**. Each vertebral artery gives off a branch to supply the cerebellum and medulla oblongata before uniting with its partner to form the **basilar artery**. The

Arteries

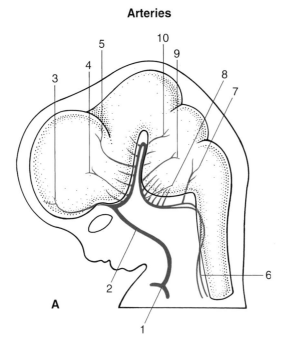

A

Veins

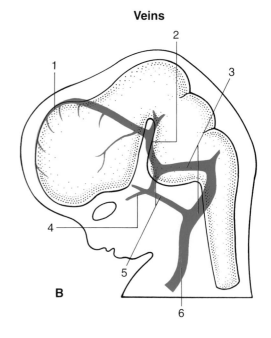

B

(A) Arteries
1. Aortic arch
2. Internal carotid
3. Anterior cerebral
4. Middle cerebral
5. Posterior cerebral
6. Vertebrals
7. Posterior inferior cerebellar
8. Basilar
9. Anterior inferior cerebellar
10. Superior cerebellar

(B) Sinuses/veins
1. Superior sagittal
2. Transverse
3. Sigmoid
4. Cavernous
5. Petrosal
6. Internal jugular vein

Figure 30.8. Blood supply of the brain at 8 weeks.

basilar gives off two pairs of arteries to the cerebellum and upper brain stem before dividing into two terminal branches that link up with the ends of the internal carotids below the midbrain. In 25% of the population, this basic arrangement is permanent, and a carotid angiogram will display the three cerebral arteries on that side. In the remainder of the population, the vertebral arteries take over the posterior cerebral arteries, in which case the arterial segment in the interval between the middle and posterior cerebral arteries becomes the **posterior communicating artery**.

Veins

The arrangement of the cranial venous system at the end of the embryonic period is shown in *Figure 30.8B*. The veins draining the brain empty into venous sinuses which develop along lines of reflection of the dura mater. The sinuses are numbered in the figure, where the adult configuration is already discernible.

MALFORMATIONS

Malformations may be considered in relation to the following, critical phases in brain development:

1. Neurulation (weeks 3 and 4).
2. Cytogenesis in the ventricular zone of the cerebral vesicles (weeks 4–16).
3. Neuronal migration, notably along radial glial cells (weeks 6–20).
4. Circulation of the cerebrospinal fluid (from week 6 onward).
5. Neuronal maturation (from week 6 onward).

Failure of Neurulation

Anencephaly ('absence of the brain', *Figure 30.9A*) is a consequence of failure of the process of neurulation at the site of the rostral neuropore. The cerebral vesicles are unable to develop in the absence of a roof, and immature neurons and glial cells form a mushroom-like excrescence which later undergoes complete degeneration.

Most anencephalic embryos abort spontaneously. If pregnancy continues to term, many are stillborn (die before birth). Those born alive seldom survive for more than a few hours. The vault of the skull is missing, and necrotic brain tissue is exposed.

Anencephaly is one of the commonest lethal congenital malformations. In different parts of the world the incidence ranges between 1 and 6 per 1000 births at or near full term.

The reason for occurrence of anencephaly is obscure. The primary fault may be in the neuroepithelium itself, or in the prechordal

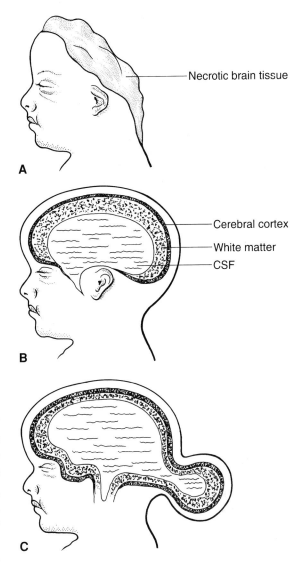

Figure 30.9. Malformations of the brain. (A) Anencephaly. (B) Hydrocephaly. (C) Hydrencephalocele.

mesoderm which supports the neural folds prior to closure of the rostral neuropore during the 4th week. The importance of dietary intake of folic acid in prevention of NTDs (neural tube defects) has been pointed out in Chapter 11. Ideally, all women should take folic acid supplements throughout the child-bearing period of life, because NTDs commence so early – during the 2nd week after the first missed menstrual period.

Failure of Cytogenesis

Sporadic occurrence of *microcephaly* ('small brain') is attributed to spontaneous gene mutation. It is a significant cause of serious mental defect, and is attributed to premature arrest of the cytogenetic phase of brain development. The cerebral cortex shows few gyri, or none (*agyria*).

Disordered Migration

Radial glial cells seem to be sensitive to *alcohol*, which passes freely from maternal to fetal blood. Current obstetric advice is to avoid alcohol totally during pregnancy, because the minimal dose required to interfere with neuronal migration is uncertain. The commonest clinical effect of chronic alcohol consumption is *mental retardation*, which becomes apparent in the early postnatal years. The commonest pathological effect is imperfect lamination of the gray matter of the cerebral cortex, apparently because of damage to the radial glial cells.

Disordered Cerebrospinal Fluid Circulation

Hydrocephaly is a quite frequent disturbance of brain development (*Figure 30.9B*). It is caused by obstruction to cerebrospinal fluid (CSF) circulation, most often by *aqueductal stenosis*. The stenosis (narrowing) is attributed to damage to the surrounding brain tissue by viral infection during the middle trimester. Passive dilatation of the lateral ventricles becomes evident on ultrasonography from the 30th week onward. Rarely, hydrocephaly is caused by failure of forma-

tion of the three apertures leading from the fourth ventricle into the subarachnoid space (*Dandy–Walker syndrome*). Another rare cause is *Arnold–Chiari malformation*, where CSF circulation is compromised by herniation of the cerebellum and medulla oblongata into the foramen magnum.

Occipital herniation is commonly associated with hydrocephaly. The simplest form is an *occipital meningocele*, consisting of an arachnoid cyst protruding through a defect in the occipital bone. (The dura mater does not protrude because it forms the endosteal lining of the skull.) If the cyst contains brain tissue, it is an *encephalocele*. If the lateral ventricle is extruded as well, it is a *hydrencephalocele* (*Figure 30.9C*).

Where meningoceles occur in the absence of ventricular dilatation, it is debatable whether the primary fault is a defect in the occipital neural arch, or is an obstruction to CSF circulation within the subarachnoid space.

Note: Some authors use the term 'hydrocephalus' for the state of the brain, and 'hydrocephaly' for the state of the affected fetus or infant.

Disordered Neuronal Maturation

Disordered maturation of neurons in the cerebral cortex causes *mental deficiency* at the intellectual level and *cerebral palsy* at the physical level. The commonest cause of these very prevalent problems, is *perfusion failure* at some time during the third trimester of pregnancy. Perfusion failure means failure to provide a sufficient amount of oxygenated blood to the fetal brain. Disordered maturation is also caused by *viral infections*, notably cytomegalovirus.

Two great causes of perfusion failure are *placental insufficiency*, and *maternal hypoten-*

sion. Both of these states can produce *fetal asphyxia.*

- Placental insufficiency can be produced by premature separation of the placenta (leading to blood loss through the vagina), or by placental infarction ('infarction' signifies necrosis of one or more placental cotyledons due to vascular thrombosis).
- Maternal hypotension can be caused by physical injury (e.g. a fall) or emotional shock (e.g. bereavement). The effect is to reduce the rate and pressure of maternal blood flow through the intervillous space, with possibly disastrous consequences for the wellbeing of the fetus.
- A third source of perfusion failure is *pulmonary insufficiency*, where the fetal lungs are underdeveloped because of prematurity (Chapter 18) or compression (Chapter 18). The risk of perfusion failure arises immediately after birth, because inadequate pulmonary ventilation leads to diminished oxygen saturation of blood in the carotid and vertebrobasilar arterial systems.

The end result of perfusion failure is an abnormally thin cerebral cortex. Patchy thinning is called *porencephaly* ('sponge brain'). Generalized thinning shortens the wavelength required for development of cortical gyri; the outcome is *polymicrogyria.* In extreme cases, the cortex is completely destroyed; the fetus/infant shows *hydranencephaly* ('water, no brain').

Note: Damage to the cerebral cortex may also occur *intranatally*, i.e. during labor. Such lesions are not classified as congenital, and are not considered here.

EMBRYOLOGICAL TERMS

Placodes. Epibranchial placodes. Ectomesenchyme. Rathke's pouch. Cortical plate. *Craniopharyngioma. Anencephaly. Microcephaly. Agyria. Hydrocephaly. Aqueductal stenosis. Dandy–Walker syndrome Arnold–Chiari malformation. Occipital meningocele. Hydrencephalocele. Porencephaly. Polymicrogyria. Hydranencephaly.*

31

Full-term placenta and fetus

It has been explained, in Chapter 3, that the placenta develops at the interface between the chorion frondosum and the decidua basalis. The chorion laeve has largely disappeared by the end of the 12th week, and the disc-like form of the placenta is established by the chorion frondosum.

FULL-TERM PLACENTA

The sites of placental attachment to the uterus have the following order of frequency: posterior wall, anterior wall, fundus. With repeated pregnancies, the blastocyst tends to descend to lower levels before it becomes attached; there is a corresponding risk of attachment to the **lower uterine segment**. The lower uterine segment is the lower part of the body of the uterus, which thins out, along with the cervix, during expulsion of the fetus at childbirth. In the case of low placental attachment, there is a danger of premature separation of the placenta during labor, with resultant antepartum hemorrhage.

Structure

When the freshly delivered placenta is examined its inner, *fetal* surface is seen to be smooth and shiny (*Figure 31.1A*), whereas the outer, *maternal* surface is rough (*Figure 31.1B*). The fetal surface is covered by the amnion, which is adherent around the placental margin and invests the umbilical cord. The umbilical vessels are visible through the amnion as they fan out from the cord before sinking into the placental substance.

The umbilical cord is 30–60 cm in length. Its gelatinous appearance is caused by a mucoid matrix embedded in extraembryonic mesoderm. The matrix is called *Wharton's jelly*. Within the cord are the two umbilical arteries, pursuing a spiral course around the single (left) umbilical vein. The allantois (*Figure 31.2*) persists within the cord for a variable period of fetal life before undergoing atrophy.

The maternal surface may show a thin film of tissue derived from the spongy layer of the decidua, sheared off the wall of the uterus during separation of the placenta. Beneath the film, this surface is divided into 15–20 irregular islands called *cotyledons*. The cotyledons are partially separated by *placental septa* projecting from the decidua basalis.

The make-up of the placenta is shown diagrammatically in *Figure 31.3*. The placental substance underlying the amnion is called the *chorionic plate*. It is made up of large fetal vessels embedded in extraembryonic meso-

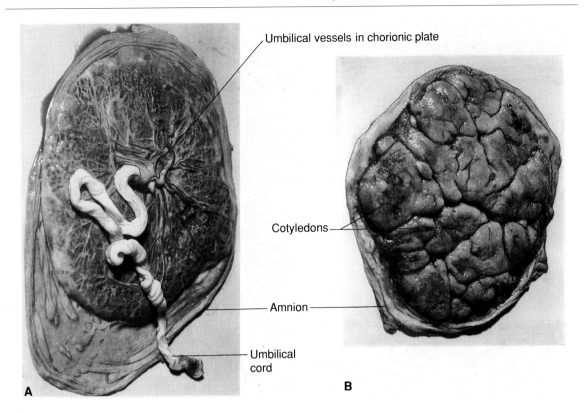

Umbilical vessels in chorionic plate

Cotyledons

Amnion

Umbilical cord

A   **B**

Figure 31.1. Full term placenta. (A) Fetal surface. (B) Maternal surface.

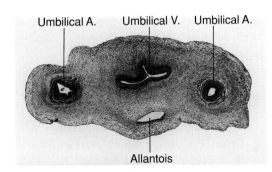

Umbilical A.   Umbilical V.   Umbilical A.

Allantois

Figure 31.2. Transverse section of the umbilical cord, at 15 weeks. (University of Washington Collection.)

derm. The decidua basalis constitutes the *basal plate*.

Some 200 villous trees emerge from the deep surface of the chorionic plate. The trees are secured to the basal plate by anchoring villi, and villous branches project into the intervillous space. The primary branches are *intermediate villi*, and the freely ending secondary or later branches are *terminal villi*. During the first trimester, much of the gaseous and nutrient exchanges between mother and fetus occur across intermediate villi (*Figure 31.4A*), whereas in the third trimester, it occurs across terminal villi (*Figure 31.4B*).

Fetal Vessels

As shown diagrammatically in *Figure 31.3*, the smaller branch arteries divide early. The arterioles that result are much more numerous than the veins, and each one breaks up to enter a capillary network. The beneficial

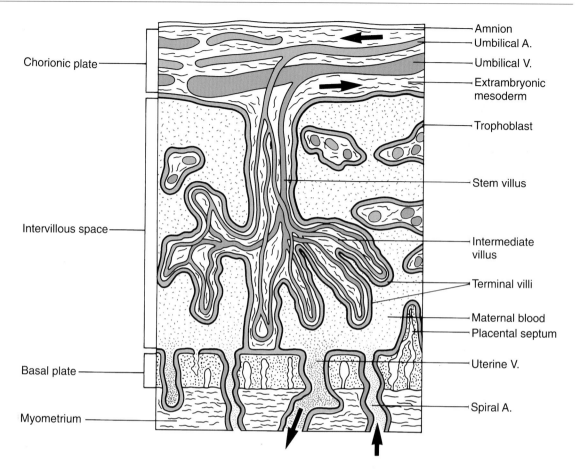

Figure 31.3. Diagrammatic section through the placenta. Red color indicates oxygenated blood; blue color indicates reduced blood. Arrows indicate directions of blood flow.

effect of this arrangement is twofold. First, it increases the size of the villous capillary bed. Secondly, it slows the rate of passage of blood into and through the capillaries, thereby permitting more complete physiological exchanges.

Placental maturation is associated with widening of individual villous capillaries, and thinning of the surface trophoblast. The cytotrophoblast is largely exhausted by the constant creation of syncytium.

Maternal Vessels

Some 200 spiral arteries discharge into the intervillous space, and about 500 ml of maternal blood pass through the intervillous space each minute. The arterial blood spurts into the intervillous space, reaching the chorionic plate before being dispersed. It returns more slowly, percolating through the villous sponge on its way to the venous exits. Gentle, rhythmic contractions of the uterus, known as *Braxton–Hicks contractions*, are thought to assist in emptying the intervillous space.

The Placental Membrane

The *placental membrane (placental barrier)* is the anatomic partition between the fetal and the maternal circulations. It is entirely of

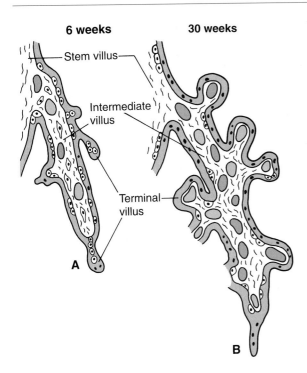

Figure 31.4. Maturation of a villous branch. (Adapted from Castellucci *et al.*)

fetal origin, having the following composition (*Figure 31.5*):

- Fetal capillary endothelium
- The basement membrane of the villus
- A film of syncytiotrophoblast.

Placental Physiology

The placenta serves four kinds of physiological function:

- as a *lung* for the function of respiratory gas exchange;
- as an *intestine* in the provision of nutrients, namely amino acids, fatty acids, sugars, minerals and vitamins;
- as a *kidney* for the elimination of the end-products of fetal metabolism;
- as an *endocrine gland* producing hormones necessary for maintenance of the pregnancy.

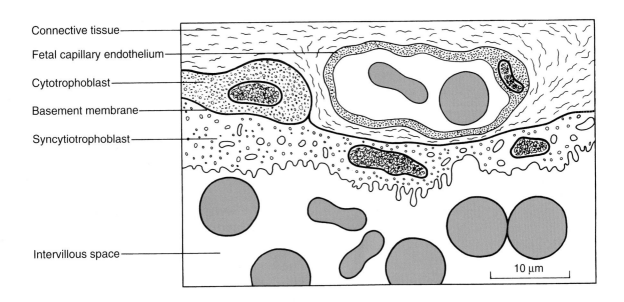

Figure 31.5. Structure of the placental membrane. All erythrocytes are colored red.

Placental Transfer Mechanisms

The placenta acts as a semipermeable membrane in permitting *diffusion* of solutes of low molecular weight, in both directions. Water, electrolytes, minerals and gases (including anesthetic gases) diffuse rapidly. The mean oxygen saturation level of the maternal blood is about 70%; the level in the tributaries of the umbilical vein is about 65%.

The relatively large molecules of steroid and peptide hormones produced by the maternal endocrine glands diffuse very slowly to the fetus.

Molecules required for nutrition of growing organs are transferred by *active transport*. Carrier molecules shuttle back and forth within the trophoblast, taking the nutrient molecules (sugars, amino acids, fatty acids) from the maternal surface to the fetal surface.

Pinocytosis by the trophoblast is the mechanism for uptake of very large molecules from the intervillous space. Gamma globulins are transferred in this way, giving the infant a passive immunity to viral infections acquired by the mother in early life (measles, rubella, whooping cough). Unfortunately, viruses themselves utilize the same mechanism: hence the fetal risk in cases of current maternal infection by rubella or AIDS. On the other hand, bacteria are not transported, and fetal bacterial infection can only occur if the placenta is damaged by bacterial inflammation.

AMNIOTIC FLUID

The normal volume of amniotic fluid at full term (end of pregnancy) is about 700 ml. During the first trimester, fluid enters the amniotic sac from outside by diffusion from the surrounding decidua, and from inside by diffusion from the embryo through the surface ectoderm. Later on, the chief sources are the fetal kidneys at a rate of about 700 ml per day, and the fetal lungs at about 350 ml per day. The composition of amniotic fluid resembles that of dilute urine.

Circulation

The amniotic fluid is in a constant state of circulation, and renewal, as follows:

1. It is swallowed by the fetus and absorbed from the intestine into the fetal blood stream.
2. Some is absorbed from the fetal blood stream, by diffusion across the placental membrane into the intervillous space.
3. Some is excreted by the fetal kidneys (and to a smaller extent by the lungs) into the amniotic sac.

Rupture of the Membranes

With the onset of labor, uterine contractions force a cone of amniotic sac into the cervical canal. The cervix responds by a progressive dilatation, whereupon the cone ruptures and a variable amount of amniotic fluid escapes (so-called 'rupture of the membranes,' or 'escape of the waters') before the cervix is plugged by the descending fetal head.

THE FETAL CIRCULATION

The fetal circulation is illustrated in *Figure 31.6*, to which the numbers in the following paragraphs refer.

The umbilical vein (1) carries oxygenated blood from the placenta to the fetus. Having

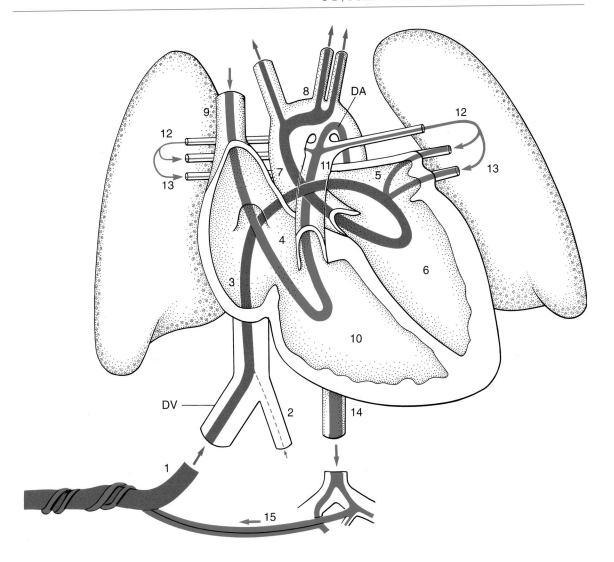

Figure 31.6. Diagram of the fetal circulation. For the numbers, see text. DA, ductus arteriosus; DV, ductus venosus.

reached the liver, almost all of the blood is shunted through the ductus venosus, to the stem of the inferior caval vein. Some deoxygenated blood is added from the lower part of the inferior caval vein (2), which is returning blood from the lower limbs and lower part of the trunk.

Having entered the right atrium (3), the blood is sent through the oval foramen (4) into the left atrium (5), and from here through the left ventricle (6) into the ascend-

ing aorta (7). The head, neck and upper limbs receive this blood through the three great vessels (8) arising from the aortic arch.

The blood returns to the heart through the superior caval vein (9). It passes through the right atrium into the right ventricle (10), and pulmonary trunk (11). A small amount enters lungs through the pulmonary arteries (12), returning to the heart in the pulmonary veins (13). The bulk enters the descending aorta (14) through the ductus arteriosus, for return to the placenta by way of the umbilical arteries (15). A small amount is distributed to the lower limbs and lower part of the trunk.

CIRCULATORY CHANGES AT BIRTH

Two events immediately following birth have a dramatic effect on the circulation:

- Blood flow ceases in the umbilical vessels, which either undergo spontaneous constriction or are clamped by the obstetrician's forceps. As a result, venous pressure in the right atrium falls to near zero.
- During the first inspiratory effort, the pulmonary vascular bed opens up and blood is diverted to the lungs. As a result, arterial pressure in the ductus arteriosus falls to near zero, and left atrial pressure rises due to massive influx of blood from the lungs.

The reversal of pressure relationships of the two atria ensures that the oval foramen is sealed off by the septum primum. Collapse of pressure in the ductus arteriosus has two effects: (a) It leads to takeover of the descending aorta (and its branches) by the output of the left ventricle. (b) Oxygenated blood leaks from the aortic arch into the ductus arteriosus. The muscle cells in the tunica media of the ductus arteriosus are uniquely sensitive to oxygen, which elicits sustained contraction of these cells.

Adherence of the septum primum to the limbus (margin) of the oval fossa is secured initially by fibrinous deposits along the line of contact. During the first postnatal year, the fibrin is replaced by fibrous connective tissue, which is also used to strengthen the interior of the septum primum.

POSTNATAL CIRCULATION

The postnatal circulaton is illustrated in *Figure 31.7*, to which the numbers in the following paragraphs refer.

From the inferior vena cava (1) and superior caval vein (2), venous blood enters the right atrium (3). The entire blood flow enters the right ventricle (4) to be sent through the pulmonary trunk (5) and pulmonary arteries (6) into the lungs.

Oxygenated blood returns via the pulmonary veins (7) to the left atrium (8) which transmits it to the left ventricle (9). Left ventricular contraction fills the ascending aorta (10) and the aortic arch, from which the great arteries to the head, neck, and upper limbs (11) are given off. Blood that bypasses these vessels enters the descending aorta (12) for distribution to the trunk and lower limbs.

Fibrous Vascular Remnants

The umbilical vein and ductus venosus are slowly replaced by fibrous tissue. Their remnants in the adult are, respectively, the **ligamentum teres**, in the free edge of the falciform ligament, and the **ligamentum venosum**, stretching from the left branch of the portal vein to the inferior caval vein. Curiously, the lumens of both remain patent throughout life.

The ductus arteriosus is represented in the adult by the **ligamentum arteriosum**, attaching the stem of the left pulmonary artery to the under surface of the aortic arch.

MALFORMATIONS

Hydramnios is a common abnormality (1 in 200 pregnancies), where the volume of

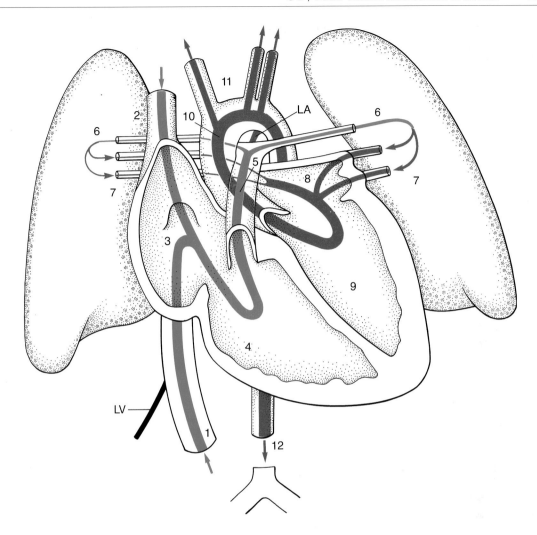

Figure 31.7. Diagram of the circulation after birth. For the numbers, see text. LA, ligamentum arteriosum; LV, ligamentum venosum.

amniotic fluid exceeds 2 liters. One case in five is associated with anencephaly. The responsible feature in anencephalics is deficient development of the fetal neuro hypophysis, with consequent diabetes insipidus. (The neurohypophysis normally secretes antidiuretic hormone, which causes large amounts of fluid to be absorbed from the distal convoluted tubules of the kidney.) Another known cause of hydramnios is atresia of the esophagus or duodenum; by pre-

venting absorption of amniotic fluid from the intestine into the fetal blood stream, this blocks the normal route of access to the intervillous space.

Oligohydramnios is a relatively rare condition where the volume of fluid amounts to less than 500 ml. The usual cause is deficient production of fetal urine, and renal malformation or urinary tract obstruction should always be suspected. An extreme example is *Potter's syndrome*, where bilateral renal agenesis is associated with virtual absence of amniotic fluid. The consequent direct pressure of the uterine wall on the fetus produces characteristic flattening of the face and distortion of the ears, along with underdevelopment of the lungs brought about by compression of the thorax.

EMBRYOLOGICAL TERMS

Wharton's jelly. Cotyledons. Placental septa. Chorionic plate. Basal plate. Intermediate, terminal villi. Placental membrane. *Hydramnios. Oligohydramnios. Potter's syndrome.*

Glossary of embryological terms

Note: Terms in *italics* denote abnormalities

abortion Expulsion of conceptus before viability (20 weeks). *Spontaneous abortion* usually occurs before 12 weeks. *Therapeutic abortion* is medically induced

abortus All of the material expelled during an abortion

acrosome reaction Liberation of acrosomal contents during penetration of corona radiata by sperm (Ch. 2)

adnexa The fetal membranes (amnion, chorion, allantois) (Ch. 31)

afterbirth Placenta plus amnion and attached chorion laeve (Ch. 31)

agenesis Nonformation of a body part, e.g. renal agenesis (Ch. 21)

agyria Absence of gyri from the cerebral cortex; a disturbance of cortical migration (Ch. 30)

alar plate Dorsal part of neural tube (Ch. 10)

allantois Endodermal diverticulum extending from yolk sac into connecting stalk (Ch. 4)

amelia Absence of one or more limbs (Ch. 12)

amnion Flat-celled membrane, attached around the margin of the epiblast (Ch. 4)

amniotic sac Vesicle enclosed by amnion and epiblast; encloses the entire embryo after completion of the body folds (Chs 4 and 5)

anal membrane Dorsal subdivision of the cloacal membrane (Ch. 23)

anal pit Depression external to anal membrane (Ch. 23)

anchoring villus Villus attached to basal plate (Ch. 3)

anencephalus Absence of the telencephalon (Ch. 30)

anencephaly Term used to signify a state of anencephalus (Ch. 30)

angioblasts Mesodermal cells that form primitive blood vessels (Ch. 7)

annular pancreas Ring-like development of pancreatic tissue around the duodenum (Ch. 19)

anomaly Term used in respect of congenital defects. 'Major anomalies' include major congenital malformations, and all of the inborn errors of metabolism. 'Minor anomalies' are relatively trivial macroscopic malformations (Ch. 1)

anorectal agenesis Collective term for maldevelopments of the rectum and anal canal (Ch. 23)

aortic arches The pharyngeal arch arteries (Ch. 13)

aortic sac Expanded distal end of truncus arteriosus (Chs 8 and 13)

aortopulmonary septum Septum dividing the truncus arteriosus into aortic and pulmonary channels (Ch. 16)

apical ectodermal ridge Ectodermal thickening at tip of limb bud (Ch. 12)

arcuate uterus Uterus with flat or concave top (no fundus) (Ch. 22)

athelia Absence of nipple(s), and therefore of breast(s) (Ch. 11)

atresia Failure of development of a body part, e.g. esophageal atresia (Ch. 18)

aural hillocks Primordia of the auricle (Chs 25 and 27)

axial artery Core artery of the limb bud (Ch. 12)

azygos lobe Part of the right upper pulmonary lobe lying medial to the azygos vein (Ch. 18)

basal plate (a) The ventrolateral plate of the neural tube (Ch. 10). Also (b) The decidua basalis at full term (Ch. 31)

bifid uvula Mildest form of cleft palate (Ch. 25)

bilaminar embryonic disc Disc composed of epiblast and hypoblast (Ch. 4)

biliary atresia Failed development of the intra-hepatic and/or extrahepatic ducts

blastemal vertebra Mesenchymal phase of vertebral development (Ch. 11)

blastomeres Cells produced by cleavage of the zygote (Ch. 2)

blastocyst Pre-implantation embryo comprising embryoblast and trophoblast (Ch. 2)

blood islands Patches of hemopoietic tissue on the wall of the yolk sac (Ch. 7)

body stalk See **connecting stalk**

brain plate Rostral part of neural plate (Ch. 5)

branchial arches See **pharyngeal arches**

branchial cyst Congenital cyst derived from the cervical sinus (Ch. 24)

branchial fistula Ruptured branchial cyst

buccopharyngeal membrane Term used to denote the oral membrane

bud Primordium, earliest rudiment

bulbus cordis Ill-defined term (not used herein), usually taken to signify the future right ventricle

capacitation Removal of a glycoprotein coat from spermatozoa, giving them the capacity to penetrate the oocyte (Ch. 2)

cardiac jelly Gelatinous subendocardial layer, giving rise to cushion tissue (Ch. 14)

cardinal veins Receive blood from the intersegmental veins; drain into the sinus venosus. (Chs 7 and 14)

cardiogenic mesoderm Mesoderm in the floor of the embryonic coelom, that forms the heart tube (Chs 7 and 14)

caudal Tailward

caudal eminence Ectodermal cells (neural cord) involved in secondary neurulation (Ch. 10)

caudal mesoderm Embryonic mesoderm caudal to the cloacal membrane (Ch. 4)

caul Midwives' term applied to an unruptured amniotic sac surrounding a newborn infant

centrum Body of blastemal vertebra (Ch. 11)

cephalic Headward

cervical flexure Flexure at junction of hindbrain with presumptive spinal cord (Ch. 29)

cervical sinus Ectoderm-lined pouch, created by fusion of hyoid arch with epipericardial ridge (Ch. 24)

chondrocranium Cartilaginous base of the fetal skull (Ch. 26)

choriocarcinoma Highly malignant trophoblastic tumor (Ch. 3)

chorion Trophoblast together with underlying extraembryonic mesoderm (Ch. 3)

chorion frondosum The 'frilly' chorion penetrating the decidua basalis (Ch. 3)

chorion laeve The smooth chorion underlying the decidua parietalis (Ch. 3)

chorionic plate Sheet of chorion on the fetal aspect of the placenta; contains branches of the umbilical vessels (Ch. 31)

chorionic sac Chorionic vesicle (Ch. 3)

chorionic vesicle The newly implanted conceptus (Ch. 3)

chorionic villi Placental villi containing blood vessels (Ch. 3)

chromosomal sex Cellular sex, based on detection of inactive X chromosome in female cells (Ch. 22)

cleavage 'Splitting.' The process of cell division whereby the zygote is converted into a morula (Ch. 2)

cleavage furrow Furrow surrounding equator of zygote, at onset of first cleavage division (Ch. 2)

cleft lip Result of failure of fusion of maxillary prominence with intermaxillary segment (Ch. 25)

cleft palate Result of failure of fusion of palatal processes (Ch. 25)

cloaca Blind, terminal portion of the hindgut

cloacal membrane Area of adhesion of ectoderm to endoderm, caudal to the primitive streak (Ch. 4)

coarctation of the aorta Congenital malformation where the aortic arch is narrowed, usually proximal to a persistent ductus arteriosus (Ch. 17)

cochlear sac Compartment of the otocyst; forms cochlear duct and saccule, with their sensory receptor epithelium (Ch. 27)

coloboma 'Keyhole' iris, due to persistence of the optic fissure (Ch. 28)

common arterial trunk Malformation resulting from agenesis of the aortopulmonary septum (Ch. 17)

common atrioventricular canal Canal leading from the common atrium to the left ventricle (Ch. 14)

common atrium Primitive heart chamber, forerunner of left and right atria (Ch. 14)

common dorsal mesentery Dorsal mesentery suspending the small and large intestines (Ch. 20)

conceptus The products of conception, namely the embryo and membranes (Ch. 1)

congenital hernial sac A persistent processus vaginalis (Ch. 22)

congenital malformation Abnormality present at birth and attributable to abnormal intrauterine development (Ch. 1)

conjoint twins Fused twins, produced by partial or complete duplication of the primitive streak (Ch. 9)

connecting stalk Stalk of extraembryonic mesoderm suspending the embryo; forerunner of the umbilical cord (Ch. 4)

conus cordis Ill-defined term (not used herein), usually taken to signify the outflow channel of the embryonic right ventricle

corona radiata cells of cumulus oophorus surrounding the secondary oocyte after ovulation (Ch. 2)

corpus albicans Scarred remnant of corpus luteum (Ch. 2)

corpus luteum Endocrine gland derived from the ruptured ovarian follicle (Ch. 2)

cortical reaction Reaction of the cortex of the oocyte, preventing penetration by more than one spermatozoon (Ch. 2)

costal process Mesenchymal rib rudiment (Ch. 11)

cotyledons Placental islands created by placental septa (Ch. 31)

cranial Headward (*cranium*, skull)

craniopharyngioma Tumor originating from Rathke's pouch (Ch. 30)

craniostenosis Premature fusion of skull sutures

crown–rump length Sitting height (Ch. 1)

cryptorchism (*cryptorchidism*) Complete failure of testicular descent (Ch. 22)

cumulus oophorus Cells of stratum granulosum surrounding the secondary oocyte prior to ovulation (Ch. 2)

cytotrophoblast Cellular layer of the trophoblast (Ch. 3)

cytotrophoblastic shell Shell of trophoblast surrounding the chorionic vesicle (Ch. 3)

decidua Endometrium of pregnancy (Ch. 3)

decidua basalis Decidua to which chorion frondosum is attached (Ch. 3)

decidua capsularis Decidua enclosing the chorionic vesicle (Ch. 3)

decidua parietalis Decidua not invaded by trophoblast (Ch. 3)

definitive oocyte Oocyte after completion of the second meiotic division. The 'egg' of lay terminology (Ch. 2)

deformation Change in shape or position of a previously normal part; mainly used with reference to temporary molding from compression, in association with oligohydramnios (Ch. 31)

dental lamina Ectodermal precursor of enamel organs (Ch. 26)

dental papilla Mesenchyme enclosed by the enamel organ; forms the dentin and the dental pulp (Ch. 26)

dental sac Fibrous shell surrounding the tooth germ (Ch. 26)

dermatome Subdivision of the somite. Forms the dermis (connective tissue layer) of the skin (Chs 8 and 11)

determination Commitment to a specific line of development

dextrocardia Heart on the right side; usually accompanied by partial or complete situs inversus (Ch. 17)

diencephalon Portion of prosencephalon flanking the third ventricle (Ch. 29)

differentiation Intracellular changes during normal development, leading to appearance of new cell types (Ch. 1)

digital rays Five mesenchymal condensations in the limb plate; forerunners of metacarpus/metatarsus and digits (Ch. 12)

dizygotic twins Fraternal twins, produced from two zygotes (Ch. 9)

dorsal Toward the back of the embryo

dorsal aortas Initially paired embryonic vessels linking the truncus arteriosus to the umbilical arteries. The pair are often called 'aortae', although this is merely a phonetic spelling of a Greek word (Ch. 7)

dorsal mesocardium Temporary dorsal mesentery, enclosing the heart tube (Ch. 14)

dorsal mesogastrium Dorsal mesentery of the stomach (Ch. 19).

dorsal pancreatic bud Primordium of the uncinate process (Ch. 19)

double aortic arch Malformation showing persistence of a right aortic arch (Ch. 17)

ductus arteriosus Channel connecting left pulmonary artery to aortic arch (Ch. 13)

ductus venosus Channel connecting (left) umbilical vein to inferior cava; contains oxygenated blood (Ch. 19)

duplex twins Fused twins, produced by partial duplication of the primitive streak (Ch. 9)

dysplasia Faulty development

ectoderm The germ layer that forms the nervous system, as well as the epidermis and its derivatives

ectopia Development in an abnormal location, e.g ectopic pregnancy (Ch. 3), ectopic kidney (Ch. 21), ectopic testis (Ch. 22)

ectopia cordis Rare malformation where the heart lies partly or completely outside the rib cage (Ch. 17)

ectopic pregnancy Pregnancy following implantation outside the cavity of the uterus (Ch. 3)

embryo The organism during the period between the beginning of the 3rd week and the end of the 8th week of development (Ch. 1)

embryology The study of prenatal development (Ch. 1)

embryonic coelom The serous cavity formed within the embryo; forerunner of the pericardial, pleural, and peritoneal sacs (Chs 4 and 8)

embryonic disc Oval, later pear-shaped early embryo, comprising two, later three, germ layers (Ch. 4)

embryonic foregut Segment of gut between oral membrane and vitelline duct (Ch. 6)

embryonic hindgut Segment of gut between vitelline duct and cloacal membrane (Ch. 6)

embryonic midgut Segment of gut facing into the vitelline duct (Ch. 6)

embryonic period First 8 weeks of development (Ch. 1)

embryonic pharynx Most rostral part of the embryonic foregut, enclosed by the pharyngeal arches

embryonic tail Caudal projection formed by 8 or 9 coccygeal vertebrae (Ch. 11)

enamel organ Ectodermal precursor of tooth enamel (Ch. 26)

endocardal cushions Swellings composed of cardiac jelly, in the wall of the common atrioventricular canal. Cushion tissue also occupies the wall of the cardiac outflow channel

endoderm The germ layer that forms the epithelium of the embryonic gut and its derivatives (Ch. 4)

epiblast Columnar epithelium lining the floor of the amniotic sac (Ch. 4)

epibranchial placodes Patches of thickened surface ectoderm overlying the pharyngeal arches; contribute sensory ganglion cells to underlying cranial nerves (Ch. 24)

epigenesis The sequence of development of body parts

epimere Dorsal subdivision of a myotome (Ch. 11)

exomphalos Congenital umbilical hernia (Ch. 20)

exstrophy of the bladder Failed development of the infraumbilical abdominal wall and anterior bladder wall

extraembryonic coelom The cavity surrounding the embryo, within the chorionic vesicle (Ch. 3)

extraembryonic mesoderm Initially, branched cells derived from the epiblast, filling the extraembryonic coelom and forming the connecting stalk (Ch. 4); later, forms the connective tissue and blood vessels within the tertiary chorionic villi (Chs 3 and 31)

female pronucleus The haploid nucleus of the oocyte at fertilization (Ch. 2)

fertilization Union of male and female gametes (Ch. 2)

fertilization age True age of the embryo/fetus, where the day of fertilization (i.e. of coitus) is known (Ch. 1)

fetal membranes Amnion, chorion and allantois (Ch. 31)

fetal period Period between beginning of week 9 of development, and full term (Ch. 1)

fetus The organism in the period between the beginning of week 9 of development, and full term (Ch. 1)

first polar body Discarded cell material following the first meiotic division (Ch. 2)

fistula Pathological channel, open at both ends

flexion Folding of the embryo (Ch. 6)

foetus Old spelling of fetus

folding Formation of the head fold, tail fold and lateral body folds (Ch.6)

follicular antrum Cavity within the ovarian follicle (Ch. 2)

follicular atresia Shrinkage and disappearance of primordial follicles during fetal life (Ch. 22)

fontanelles Temporary membranous areas of the skull, prior to fusion of the bones (Ch. 26)

foramen ovale Oval foramen in the heart (Ch. 15)

foramen primum 'First foramen' in the septum primum (Ch. 15)

foramen secundum 'Second foramen' in septum primum (Ch. 15)

foregut *Embryonic foregut* extends from oral membrane to vitelline duct opening; *definitive foregut* extends from lower end of esophagus to point of entry of bile duct (Ch. 19)

fossa ovalis Oval fossa in the heart

frontonasal prominence Mesenchymal swelling in upper facial region (Ch. 25)

gamete Mature male or female sex cell (Ch. 2)

gastrulation The process of invagination resulting in formation of the three germ layers (Ch. 4)

genital swellings Mesodermal swellings lateral to the urogenital folds; precursors of the scrotum in males and of the labia majora in females (Ch. 23)

germ cells Gametes

germ layers The ectoderm, mesoderm and endoderm (Ch. 4)

gestation Pregnancy

gestational age Embryonic/fetal age calculated from the first day of the last menstrual period before conception; exceeds developmental age by about 2 weeks (Ch. 1)

genotypic sex Chromosomal sex

glioblasts Precursors of neuroglial cells (Ch. 10)

gonadal ridge Ridge on the medial aspect of the mesonephros; precursor of the gonad (Ch. 22)

granulosa lutein cells Cells of the corpus luteum, secreting progesterone (Ch. 2)

gravid Pregnant

gubernaculum Mesenchymal strand connecting the gonad to the lower abdominal wall (Ch. 22)

gut Endodermal tube extending from oral membrane to cloacal membrane; ultimately, the endoderm forms the epithelial lining of the alimentary tract

hand plate Hand primordium (Ch. 12)

head fold The rostral body fold (Ch. 6)

head mesenchyme Diffuse, mesenchymal investment of the developing brain (Ch. 24)

hemimelia Absence of a segment of a limb (Ch. 12)

hemocytoblasts Hemopoietic stem cells (Ch. 7)

hepatic diverticulum See **liver bud**

hermaphrodite Individual possessing an ovary and a testis

Heuser's membrane Temporary membrane enclosing the primary yolk sac (Ch. 4)

hindgut Segment of embryonic gut extending from opening of vitelline duct to cloacal membrane (Ch. 6)

Hirschsprung's disease A cause of large bowel obstruction, characterized by an aganglionic segment in the distal hindgut (Ch. 23)

histogenesis Development of a tissue

horseshoe kidneys Kidneys with lower poles fused across the midline (Ch. 21)

hyaloid vessels Blood vessels supplying the lens at first; later, become the central vessels of the retina (Ch. 28)

hydatidiform mole Benign tumor composed of edematous chorionic villi (Ch. 3)

hydranencephaly Total destruction of the cerebral cortex due to perfusion failure (Ch. 30)

hydrencephalocele Brain hernia containing part of one or both lateral ventricles (Ch. 30)

hydrocele Collection of fluid within the tunica vaginalis

hydrocephaly Abnormal accumulation of cerebrospinal fluid within the ventricular system and/or subarachnoid space (Ch. 30)

hyoid arch Second pharyngeal arch (Ch. 24)

hypoblast Cuboidal epithelium underlying the epiblast (Ch. 4)

hypomere Ventral subdivision of a myotome (Ch. 11)

hypopharyngeal eminence Primordium of posterior one-third of the tongue (Ch. 24)

hypospadias Malformation where the urethra opens on the under surface of the penis (Ch. 23)

imperforate anus A form of anorectal agenesis; the anal canal is separated from the rectum by a tissue diaphragm (Ch. 23)

implantation The embedding of the blastocyst in the endometrium (Ch. 3)

incomplete descent of testis Failure of a testis to complete its migration to the scrotum (Ch. 22).

induction Stimulation of a competent tissue to develop in a particular direction

inguinal fold Fold connecting gonad to ventral body wall; contains the gubernaculum (Ch. 22)

intermaxillary segment Block of mesoderm in the interval between the maxillary prominences (Ch. 25)

intermediate mesoderm Unsegmented mesoderm in the interval between paraxial and lateral plate mesoderm (Ch. 5)

intermediate villi Primary branches of anchoring villi (Ch. 31)

intersegmental arteries and veins Vessels passing between the somites to supply the somites and neural tube. Main derivatives are the intercostal and lumbar vessels. (Chs 7 and 11)

interventricular foramen Communication between the embryonic ventricles of the heart (Ch. 16)

intervillous space Labyrinthine space within which chorionic villi are suspended; contains maternal blood (Chs 3 and 31)

isomerism Mirror-image development of body parts

karyotype Chromosomal constitution of a cell, as seen in squash preparations

labioscrotal folds Paired folds that form the labia majora (female) or scrotum (male) (Ch. 23). Synonymous with genital swellings.

lacunae Blood-filled spaces created by erosion of maternal sinusoids by the trophoblast (Ch. 3)

lanugo The first, fine coat of body hair (Ch. 11)

laryngotracheal groove Midline groove in the floor of the foregut; forerunner of the lower respiratory tract (Ch. 18)

laryngotracheal tube Tube formed from the laryngotracheal groove (Ch. 18)

lateral body folds Folds formed on each side of the flexing embryo (Ch. 6)

lens placode Ectodermal precursor of the lens vesicle (Ch. 28)

lens vesicle Hollow sphere formed from the lens placode; precursor of the lens (Ch. 28)

limb buds Outgrowths of body wall that form the limbs. (Ch. 12)

lingual swellings Paired primordia of the anterior two-thirds of the tongue (Ch. 24)

liquor folliculi Fluid within antrum of ovarian follicle

liver bud Endodermal diverticulum that forms the hepatobiliary apparatus (Ch. 19)

lung buds Endodermal buds arising from the respiratory diverticulum (Ch. 18)

maldescent of testis Testis lying outside its normal pathway of descent, e.g. in the thigh (Ch. 22)

male pronucleus Haploid nucleus of the sperm following penetration of the definitive oocyte (Ch. 2)

mammary ridge thickening of surface ectoderm, along a line extending from axilla to groin; gives rise to mammary gland (Ch. 11)

mandibular arch First pharyngeal arch (Ch. 24)

maxillary prominence Mandibular arch mesenchyme extending rostral to stomodeum (Chs 24 and 25)

meatal atresia Failure of canalization of the external acoustic meatus (Ch. 27)

meatal plate Temporary ectodermal plug in external acoustic meatus (Ch. 27)

Meckel's cartilage Cartilaginous core of the mandibular arch

Meckel's diverticulum A blind pocket projecting from the ileum, near the ileocaecal junction; remnant of vitelline duct (Ch. 20)

meconium Intestinal content during the second half of gestation

median thyroid rudiment Midline endodermal outgrowth, later marked by the foramen cecum (Ch. 24)

meningocele Spina bifida aperta, with a meningeal cyst containing only cerebrospinal fluid (Ch. 11)

meningoencephalocele Meningeal cyst containing part of the brain (Ch. 30)

meningomyelocele As above, except that the cyst contains nerve roots or spinal cord (Ch. 11)

menstrual age Gestation time, counted from the first day of the last menstrual period (Ch. 1) *meromelia* Failed development of a proximal limb segment (Ch. 12)

mesectoderm Mesenchymal cells derived from the neural crest (Ch. 10)

mesencephalon Midbrain vesicle (Ch. 29)

mesenchyme Loose embryonic mesoderm

mesoderm Middle layer of the trilaminar embryonic disc; forms connective tissues, cardiovascular system, striated and smooth muscles (Ch. 4)

mesoesophagus A dorsal mesentery suspending the lower part of the esophagus; becomes incorporated into the diaphragm (Ch. 18)

mesonephric duct Forerunner of the ductus deferens (Chs 21 and 22)

mesonephros Temporary kidney. In males, mesonephric tubules form the duct system of the testis. (Chs 21 and 22)

metanephric cap Condensation of intermediate mesoderm around the ureteric bud; forms the nephrons (Ch. 21)

metanephros Permanent kidney

microcephaly Premature fusion of skull sutures associated with underdevelopment of the brain (Chs 26 and 30)

micrognathia Abnormally small mandible (Ch. 26)

midbrain flexure Flexure at the level of the mesencephalon (Ch. 29)

midgut Initially, the embryonic gut facing into the vitelline duct; later, the territory of the superior mesenteric artery (mid-duodenum to splenic flexure of colon) (Chs 6 and 20)

miscarriage Spontaneous abortion

monozygotic twins Identical twins, produced from a single zygote (Ch. 9)

morphogen Organizing factor that determines the developmental pathway to be followed by a particular cell group

morphogenesis The process of development of form and size

morula 'Mulberry' of cells produced by the process of cleavage (Ch. 2)

Mullerian duct Paramesonephric duct (Ch. 22)

mutation Heritable change in gene structure

myelocele Spina bifida aperta, with open neural plate (Ch. 11)

myeloschisis 'Split marrow,' i.e. ununited neural folds; alternative name for myelocele

myelon 'Marrow' of vertebral column, i.e. spinal cord

myotome Subdivision of the somite. Myotomes form the skeletal muscles of the trunk; also the lingual muscles. (Chs 8 and 11)

nasal capsule Cartilaginous capsule enclosing the olfactory sense organ; forerunner of the ethmoid bone (Ch. 26)

nasal pit Recess created by the nasal prominences; nasal placode is in its roof (Ch. 25)

nasal prominences Extensions of the frontonasal prominence (Ch. 25)

nasal sac Expansion of the nasal pit; roofed by olfactory epithelium (Ch. 25)

nasolacrimal furrow Groove extending from inner angle of the eye, to the nasal sac; forerunner of the nasolacrimal duct (Ch. 25)

neonatal period The first 4 weeks after birth

neural arch Mesenchymal arch surrounding the neural tube (Ch. 11)

neural cord Precursor of the caudal end of the neural tube (Ch. 10)

neural crest Initially, crest of neural fold; later, ribbon of ectodermal epithelium dorsolateral to the neural tube (Ch. 5)

neural folds Paired folds arising from the neural plate (Ch. 5)

neural groove Midline groove between the two neural folds (Ch. 5)

neural plate Slipper-shaped ectodermal thickening in the floor of the amniotic sac; forerunner of the nervous system (Ch. 5)

neural tube Ectodermal tube formed by union of the two neural folds; forms the nervous system (Ch. 5)

neurenteric canal Temporary passage from yolk sac into amniotic sac, through the primitive node (Ch. 4)

neuroepithelial cells Cells forming the walls of the neural tube (Ch. 10)

neurulation Process whereby the neural tube is formed from the neural plate (Ch. 5)

neuropores Temporary openings at each end of the neural tube (Ch. 5)

nondisjunction Failure of a homologous pair of chromosomes to separate during meiosis; results in trisomy of the zygote upon fertilization (Ch. 1)

notochord Rod-like rostral extension from the primitive node (Ch. 4)

notochordal process Hollow rod extending rostrally from the primitive node (Ch. 4)

notochordal plate Rod-like rostral extension from the primitive streak, incorporated temporarily into the endoderm (Ch. 4)

occipital sclerotomes Sclerotomes derived from occipital somites; form neural arches around the hindbrain (Ch. 26)

oligohydramnios Deficiency of amniotic fluid (Ch. 31)

ontogeny The complete developmental history of the individual

oogonia Female primordial germ cells (Ch. 22)

optic cup Invaginated optic vesicle (Ch. 28)

optic fissure Fissure extending along under surface of optic cup and stalk; contains hyaloid vessels (Ch. 28)

optic groove Groove in side wall of diencephalon; lining neurectoderm forms the retina (Ch. 28)

optic outgrowth Intermediate phase of growth, between optic groove and optic vesicle phases (Ch. 29)

optic stalk Extension of the neural tube, attaching optic vesicle to diencephalon; forerunner of the optic nerve (Ch. 28)

optic vesicle Vesicle formed from the neuroepithelium lining the optic groove; forerunner of the retina (Chs 8 and 29)

oral membrane Patch of adhesion of ectoderm to endoderm, rostral to notochord (Ch. 4)

organogenesis Formation of an organ by assembly of tissues of different kinds

oropharyngeal membrane Oral membrane

otic capsule Cartilaginous capsule enclosing the membranous labyrinth (Ch. 26)

otic placode Patch of thickened ectoderm beside the hindbrain; primordium of the otocyst (Ch. 27)

otic vesicle Otocyst (Ch. 27)

otocyst Cyst derived from the otic placode; precursor of the inner ear (Ch. 27)

outflow channel Channel leading from the embryonic right ventricle to the aortic sac (Ch. 14)

oval foramen (foramen ovale) Foramen enclosed by septum secundum (Ch. 15)

ovulation Expulsion of the secondary oocyte from the ovarian follicle, into the peritoneal cavity (Ch. 2)

ovum Ill-defined term (not used herein); usually refers to secondary oocyte

palatal shelves Projections of maxillary mesoderm into the oral cavity; fuse with the primary palate to complete the secondary palate (Ch. 25)

parachordal cartilages Cartilages alongside the rostral end of the notochord; become incorporated into the basiocciput (Ch. 26)

paramesonephric ducts Paired ducts formed in the intermediate mesoderm, beside the mesonephric ducts; form the epithelial lining of the uterine tube, uterus and upper vaginal canal (Ch. 22)

paraxial mesoderm Embryonic mesoderm alongside the notochord; undergoes segmentation to form the somites (Ch. 5)

pars venosa of right atrium Part of right atrium formed from sinus venosus (Ch. 15)

parturition Birth

pelvic kidney A kidney that fails to ascend from the pelvis during development (Ch. 21)

pericardial coelom Portion of the embryonic coelom astride the midline, rostral to the oral membrane; forerunner of the pericardial cavity (Ch. 5)

periderm Superficial layer of surface ectoderm; replaced by epidermis (Ch. 11)

perinatal period The third trimester and first postnatal week

periotic capsule Shell of chondrified mesoderm surrounding the membranous labyrinth; forms the bony labyrinth (Ch. 27)

peritoneal coelom Portion of the embryonic coelom on each side, caudal to the level of the septum transversum; forerunner of peritoneal cavity (Ch. 5)

perivitelline space Interval between oocyte and zona pellucida (Ch. 2)

persistent ductus arteriosus Ductus arteriosus that remains patent after birth (Ch. 17)

phallus Precursor of penis or clitoris (Ch. 23)

pharyngeal arches Paired mesodermal thickenings in the wall of the pharynx. Derivatives include skeletal and muscular components of the face, jaws, larynx and pharynx (Ch. 24)

pharyngeal clefts Ectodermal grooves between successive pharyngeal arches (Ch. 24)

pharyngeal pouches Endodermal pockets between successive pharyngeal arches (Ch. 24)

pharynx The *embryonic pharynx* reaches from the oral membrane to the level of origin of the laryngotracheal diverticulum. The *definitive pharynx* reaches from the posterior nasal apertures to the commencement of the esophagus. (Chs 8 and 24)

phenotypic sex Sexual appearances of external genitalia

phimosis Congenital narrowing of the prepuce (Ch. 23)

phylogeny The study of ancestors in the line of evolution

physiological hernia of the midgut Extrusion of midgut into umbilical cord during the 5th to 10th weeks (Ch. 20)

placenta Organ of fetomaternal gaseous and metabolic exchange (Ch. 31)

placenta praevia Placenta attached to the lower uterine segment and/or cervix (Ch. 31)

placental membrane Partition between fetal and maternal blood (Ch. 31)

placental septa Non-eroded decidual partitions, dividing the placenta into cotyledons (Ch. 31)

placodes Thickened patches of cranial surface ectoderm. Derivatives include the lens, the membranous labyrinth and sensory ganglion cells of cranial nerves. (Ch. 29)

pleuropericardial fold Fold containing the common cardinal vein (Ch. 18)

pleuroperitoneal canal A coelomic duct, leading from the pericardial coelom to the peritoneal coelom on each side; forerunner of the pleural cavity (Ch. 5)

pleuroperitoneal membrane Shelf of somatic mesoderm, projecting into the coelom opposite the septum transversum (Ch. 18)

polar bodies Minute cells extruded from the oocyte during meiosis (Ch. 2)

polycystic kidneys Malformed kidneys, largely replaced by cysts (Ch. 21)

polymastia Supernumerary breasts (Ch. 11)

polymicrogyria Presence of innumerable, tiny gyri in the cerebral cortex, consequent to prenatal perfusion failure (Ch. 30)

polythelia Supernumerary nipples (Ch. 11)

pontine flexure Flexure within the rhombencephalon (Ch. 29)

prechordal cartilages Embryonic cartilages beneath the forebrain; form crista galli and perpendicular plate of ethmoid (Ch. 26)

prechordal plate Thickened endoderm rostral to the notochordal process; becomes part of the oral membrane (Ch. 4)

pre-embryonic period Term sometimes used to signify the first 2 weeks after fertilization

preimplantation period The interval between fertilization and implantation (Ch. 2)

presumptive atria Parts of the definitive atria formed from the common atrium (Ch. 14)

presumptive ventricles Earliest heart chambers, will form the trabeculated parts of the definitive ventricles (Ch. 14)

primary brain vesicles The forebrain, midbrain and hindbrain vesicles (Chs 8 and 29)

primary (cardiac) fold Fold formed by buckling of the heart tube (Ch. 14)

primary interventricular foramen Foramen connecting the presumptive ventricles, in the interval between the primitive interventricular foramen and the primary fold (Ch. 14)

primary interventricular septum Septum separating the presumptive (trabeculated) ventricles (Ch. 14)

primary oocyte Oocyte prior to the first meiotic division (Ch. 2)

primary palate Portion of palate formed from intermaxillary segment; forerunner of premaxilla (Ch. 25)

primary villus Villus composed only of trophoblast (Ch. 3)

primary yolk sac Temporary vesicle enclosed by Heuser's membrane and the endoderm (Ch. 4)

primitive Earliest formed, e.g. primitive ventricle

primitive dorsal mesentery Midline septum of splanchnic mesoderm, suspending the embryonic gastrointestinal tract

primitive node Expanded rostral end of primitive streak (Ch. 4)

primitive pulmonary vein Single embryonic vein draining the capillary plexuses surrounding both lung buds (Ch. 15)

primitive streak Linear zone of cell migration from the epiblast, forming the embryonic mesoderm and endoderm (Ch. 4)

primordial follicles Earliest ovarian follicles (Ch. 22)

primordial germ cell Earliest precursor of the gamete (Ch. 22)

primordium The first indication of an organ or tissue; a rudiment or bud; an *anlage* (German, pleural, *anlagen*)

processus vaginalis Pocket of peritoneum overlying the gubernaculum (Ch. 22)

proctodeum Term used by some authors for the anal pit

progress zone Mitotic mesoderm deep to apical ectodermal ridge (Ch. 12)

pronephros Earliest, temporary kidney rudiment (Ch. 21)

prosencephalon Forebrain vesicle

prospermatogonia Male primordial germ cells (Ch. 22)

pseudohermaphrodite Individual having genotypic and phenotypic sexual characters in conflict (Ch. 23)

pupillary membrane Temporary mesenchymal web overlying the pupil (Ch. 28)

quickening Perception of fetal movements by the mother, from week 16–20 onward

rachischisis Myelocele

Rathke's pouch Primordium of anterior and middle lobes of hypophysis (Ch. 30)

renal agenesis Failure of one or both kidneys to develop (Ch. 21)

respiratory diverticulum Primordium of the lungs (Ch. 18)

reversal Reversal of relationships brought about by folding of the embryo (Ch. 6)

rhombencephalon Hindbrain vesicle (Ch. 29)

rhombic lip Margin of alar plate, of rostral portion of rhombencephalon (Ch. 29)

rostral Toward the future headward end; within the head, toward the front

rostral mesoderm Embryonic mesoderm rostral to the oral membrane (Ch. 4)

rupture of the membranes Rupture of the amniotic sac at the onset of labor (Ch. 31)

sclerotome Subdivision of the somite. Two somite pairs contribute to each blastemal vertebra. (Chs 8 and 11)

secondary neurulation Formation of the lower end of the spinal cord from cells of the neural cord (Ch. 10)

secondary palate Mesodermal shelf produced by union of primary palate with the palatal shelves (Ch. 25)

secondary villus Villus composed of trophoblast with core of extraembryonic mesoderm (Ch. 4)

secondary yolk sac Endoderm-lined cavity formed from the primary yolk sac; called, simply, the yolk sac (Ch. 4)

segmentation Formation of the somites from the paraxial mesoderm (Ch. 5)

septum primum 'First septum' dividing the common atrium (Ch. 15)

septum secundum 'Second septum' dividing the common atrium (Ch. 15)

septum transversum Mesodermal septum, taking up a position between pericardial coelom and vitelline duct; forerunner of the ventral mesogastrium and of the central part of the diaphragm (Chs 5 and 18)

sex cords Columns of epithelial cells in the gonad, enclosing primordial germ cells (Ch. 22)

sexual dimorphism Development of sex differences between male and female gonads (Ch. 22)

Siamese twins A class of conjoint twins (Ch. 9)

sinual tubercle Tubercle on dorsal wall of urogenital sinus, formed by caudal ends of the paramesonephric ducts (Ch. 22)

sinuatrial (sinoatrial) orifice Opening from sinus venosus into the common atrium (Ch. 14)

sinus venosus Embryonic heart chamber receiving the main embryonic veins and opening into the common atrium (Chs 7 and 13)

situs inversus viscerum Mirror-image arrangement of thoracic and abdominal organs (Ch. 20)

somatic mesoderm Portion of lateral plate mesoderm, lateral to the embryonic coelom (Ch. 5)

somatopleure Term often used for the somatic mesoderm together with the overlying ectoderm

somite period Day 20 to day 30 of development (Ch. 5)

somites Segmental cell blocks formed from paraxial mesoderm (Ch. 5)

sperm Spermatozoon

spina bifida 'Bifid' vertebrae caused by failure of union of the neural arches in the dorsal midline (Ch. 11)

splanchnic mesoderm Portion of lateral plate mesoderm, medial to the embryonic coelom (Ch. 5)

splanchnopleure Term often used for the splanchnic mesoderm, together with the underlying endoderm

spontaneous abortion Expulsion of pre-viable conceptus without medical or mechanical aid

staging A system of classification of embryos, based on the level of development of component parts (Ch. 1)

stenosis Narrowing, e.g. pulmonary stenosis (Ch. 17)

sternal bars Paired mesenchymal rudiments which fuse to form the mesenchymal sternum (Ch. 11)

stomodeum Ectoderm-lined depression external to the oral membrane

subendocardial tubercles Synonym for endocardial cushions (Ch. 15)

stratum granulosum Epithelial cells within the ovarian follicle (Ch. 2)

succenturiate lobe Accessory lobe of the placenta (Ch. 31)

sulcus limitans Groove between alar and basal plates (Ch. 10)

syncytiotrophoblast Syncytial layer of trophoblast (Ch. 3)

syndactyly Incomplete separation of the fingers (Ch. 12)

tail fold The caudal body fold (Ch. 6)

talipes Club foot (Ch. 12)

telencephalon Embryonic cerebral hemisphere (Ch. 29)

teratogen Environmental agent capable of inducing malformation(s) in susceptible embryos (Ch. 1)

teratology The study of malformations (Ch. 1)

teratoma Tumor containing tissues derived from more than one germ layer (Ch. 4)

terminal villi Terminal branches of intermediate villi (Ch. 31)

tertiary villus Villus containing blood vessels (Ch. 3)

testicular cords Male sex cords (Ch. 22)

tetralogy of Fallot A distinctive cardiac malformation (Ch. 17)

theca lutein cells Cellular shell enclosing the corpus luteum; secretes estrogen (Ch. 2)

thyroid diverticulum Midline endodermal bud and stalk, in the interval between embryonic pharynx and aortic sac; forerunner of thyroid gland (Ch. 24)

tooth bud Enamel organ surrounding a dental papilla (Ch. 26)

tooth germ Dental sac with enclosed tooth bud (Ch. 26)

trilaminar embryonic disc Disc-shaped plate composed of the three germ layers (Ch. 4)

trimester A three calendar-month period; prenatal life is divisible into three trimesters of roughly 13 weeks each

trophoblast Initially, the cells lining the wall of the blastocyst; later, these cells erode the endometrium and line the intervillous space (Ch. 3)

trisomy Chromosomal anomaly resulting from fertilization where one gamete contains two sets of a particular chromosome, as a result of nondisjunction during meiosis (Ch. 1)

truncus arteriosus The outflow channel of the embryonic heart (Chs 7 and 13)

tubal pregnancy Pregnancy within a uterine tube (Ch. 3)

tuberculum impar Median tongue rudiment (Ch. 24)

tubotympanic recess Blind outgrowth from first pharyngeal pouch; primordium of auditory tube and tympanic cavity (Chs 24 and 27)

umbilical artery and vein Vessels linking the dorsal aorta to the placenta. The paired artery carries reduced blood, the (left) vein returns with oxygenated blood (Ch. 31)

umbilical cord The vascular connection between fetus and placenta (Chs 6 and 31)

ureteric bud Outgrowth from mesonephric duct; forms ureter, calices and collecting ducts of kidney (Ch. 21)

urethral groove Precursor of spongy urethra in males; of vestibule in females (Ch. 23)

urogenital folds Mesodermal folds flanking the urethral groove; form spongy urethra in males, labia minora in females (Ch. 23)

urogenital membrane Ventral subdivision of the cloacal membrane (Ch. 23)

urogenital ridge Mesonephros together with genital ridge (Ch. 22)

urogenital septum Coronal partition containing the paramesonephric ducts; in females, forms the broad ligament of the uterus (Ch. 23)

urogenital sinus Ventral subdivision of the cloaca (Ch. 23)

urorectal septum Mesodermal septum dividing the cloaca into urogenital sinus and rectum (Ch. 23)

vaginal plate Cell column derived from sinual tubercle (Ch. 23)

velamentous insertion of the cord Attachment of the umbilical cord to the fetal membranes beyond the placental margin (Ch. 31)

vellus Coarser hair which replaces lanugo after birth (Ch. 11)

venous valves Valves guarding the sinuatrial orifice (Ch. 15)

ventral Toward the front; equivalent to 'anterior' of gross anatomy

ventral mesogastrium Septum passing from stomach to ventral abdominal wall; derived from septum transversum (Ch. 19)

ventral pancreatic bud Outgrowth from dorsal aspect of duodenum; forerunner of entire pancreas except uncinate process (Ch. 19)

ventricular loop U-shaped loop formed by the presumptive ventricles of the heart (Ch. 14)

ventricular zone Mitotic zone of neuroepithelial cells, next to the neural canal (Ch. 10)

vernix caseosa Cheesy covering of newborn, consisting of periderm and sebaceous secretion (Ch. 11)

vestibular sac Compartment of the otocyst; forms the semicircular ducts and utricle, and their sensory receptor epithelium (Ch. 27)

viability Capacity for survival *ex utero*

vitelline arteries and veins Vessels supplying the wall of the yolk sac; become the three unpaired arteries supplying the gastrointestinal tract, and the hepatic portal system of veins (Chs 7 and 20).

Wharton's jelly Mucoid matrix of umbilical cord (Ch. 31)

Wolffian See **mesonephric**

yolk sac Synonymous with secondary yolk sac (Ch. 4)

zona pellucida Hyaline layer around the oocyte (Ch. 2)

zygote Diploid cell formed by union of male and female gametes

BASIC CONCEPTS

Babu A and Hirschhorn K (1992) A guide to human chromosome defects. *Birth Defects Original Article Series* 28: 1–18.

Brent RL (1989) The effect of embryonic and fetal exposure to X-ray, microwave and ultrasound. In *Seminars in Oncology*, vol. 16, pp. 347–368. New York: Alan R. Liss.

England MA (1983) *A Colour Atlas of Life Before Birth*. London: Wolfe Medical Publications Ltd.

Gasser RF (1975) *Atlas of Human Embryos*. Hagerstown, MD: Harper & Row.

Hall JG (1992) Developmental defects in stillborn and newborn infants. In *Developmental Pathology of the Embryo and Fetus* (Eds Dimmick JE and Kalousek DK), pp. 83–110. Philadelphia: Lippincott.

McCusick VA (1990) *Mendelian Inheritance in Man*, 9th edn. Baltimore: Johns Hopkins University Press.

Nomina embryologica (1989). In *Nomina Anatomica*, 6th edn. Edinburgh: Churchill Livingstone.

O'Rahilly R and Muller F (1987) Stages in early human development. In *Future Aspects in Human in vitro Fertilization* (Eds Feitinger W and Kemeter P). Berlin: Springer-Verlag.

O'Rahilly R and Muller F (1992) *Human Embryology and Teratology*. New York: Wiley-Liss.

FERTILIZATION, CLEAVAGE

Fredericks CM, Paulson JD and De Cherney JH (1987) *Foundations of in vitro fertilization*. Washington: Hemisphere.

Johnson M and Everitt B (1988) *Essential Reproduction*. Oxford: Blackwell.

Van Blerkom J and Motta PM (Eds) (1989) *Ultrastructure of Human Gametogenesis and Early Embryogenesis*. Boston: Kluwer.

Wolf DP and Lanzendorf SE (1991) Fertilization in man. In *A Comparative Overview of Mammalian Fertilization* (Eds Dunbar BS and O'Rand MG), pp. 385–400. New York: Plenum Press.

IMPLANTATION

Bulmer JN and Johnson PM (1990) Immunology of human placental trophoblast membrane antigens. *Arch Immunol Ther Exp* 38: 103–110.

Castellucci M, Scheper M, Scheffen I, Celona A and Kaufmann P (1990) The development of the human placental villous tree. *Anat Embryol* 181: 117–128.

Kalousek DK and Lau AE (1992) Pathology of spontaneous abortion. In *Developmental Pathology of the Embryo and Fetus* (Eds Dimmick JE and Kalousek DK), pp. 55–82. Philadelphia: Lippincott.

Roger JC and Drake BL (1987) The enigma of the fetal graft. *Am Sci* 75: 51–57.

MULTIPLE PREGNANCY

Baldwin VJ (1992) Pathology of multiple pregnancy. In *Developmental Pathology of the Fetus and Newborn* (Eds Dimmick JE and Kalousek DK), pp. 320–340. Philadelphia: Lippincott.

Spencer R (1992) Conjoined twins: theoretical embryological basis. *Teratology* 45: 591–602.

SPINAL CORD AND VERTEBRAL COLUMN

Christ B and Wilting J (1992) From somites to vertebral column. *Ann Anat* 174: 23–32

Le Douarin NM, Dupin E, Baroffio A and Dulac C (1992) New insights into the development of neural crest derivatives. *Int Rev Cytol* 138: 269–314.

Lemire RJ and Beckwith JB (1984) The spectrum of neural tube defects of the caudal spine in infants. In *The Developing Brain and its Disorders* (Eds Arima M, Suzuki Y and Yabuuchi H), pp. 29–42. Tokyo: University Press.

O'Rahilly R, Muller F and Mayer DB (1980, 1983, 1990) The human vertebral column at the end of the embryonic period proper. *J Anat* 131: 567–575, 136: 181-195, 168: 81–111.

Purves D and Lichtman JU (1985) *Principles of Neural Development*. Sunderland, MA: Sinauer.

LIMBS

Kelley RO, Fallon JF and Kelly RE (1984) Vertebrate limb morphogenesis. *Issues Rev Teratol* 2: 219–265.

O'Rahilly R (1985) The development and classification of anomalies of the limbs in the human. In *Prevention of Physical and Mental Congenital Defects. Part C: Basic and Medical Science, Education, and Future Strategies*, pp. 85–90. New York: Alan R Liss.

THORAX

Bartelings MM (1991) *The Outflow Tract of the Heart: Embryologic and Morphologic Correlations*. Holland: Proefschrift Leiden, de la Cruz Sanchez, Gomez C and Cayre R (1991) The developmental components of the ventricles: their significance in congenital heart malformations. *Cardiol Young* 1: 123–128.

Lamers WH, Wessels A, Verbeek FJ, Moorman AFM, Viragh S, Wenink ACG, Gittenbergerger-de Groot AC and Anderson RH (1992) New findings concerning ventricular septation in the human heart: implications for maldevelopment. *Circulation* 86: 1194–1205.

Moreno CN and Iovanne BA (1993) Congenital diaphragmatic hernia. *Neonatal Network* 12: 21–28

Pexieder T, Wenink ACG and Anderson RH (1989) A suggested nomenclature for the developing heart. *Int J Cardiol* 25: 255–264.

Takamura K, Okishima T, Ohdo S and Hayakawa K (1990) Association of cephalic neural crest cells with cardiovascular development, particularly that of the semilunar valves. *Anat Embryol* 182: 263–272.

Taylor GP (1992) Cardiovascular system. In *Developmental Pathology of the Embryo and Fetus* (Eds Dimmick JE and Dalousek DK), pp. 467–508. Philadelphia: Lippincott.

Thurlbeck WM (1992) Prematurity and the developing lung. Clin Perinatol 19: 497-519.

Torday J (1992) Cellular timing and fetal lung development. *Sem Perinatol* 116: 130–139.

Wigglesworth JS (1988) Lung development during the second trimester. *Brit Med Bull* 44: 894–908.

ABDOMEN, PELVIS

Bard JBL and Woolf AS (1992) Nephrogenesis and the development of renal disease. *Nephrol Dial Transplant* 7: 563–572

deVries PA and Friedland GW (1974) The staged sequential development of the anus and rectum in human embryos and fetuses. *J Pediat Surg* 9: 755–769.

FitzGerald MJT (1971) The formation of the ascending colon. *Ir J Med Sci* 140: 258–262.

FitzGerald MJT, Nolan J and O'Neill MN (1971) The position of the human caecum in fetal life. *J Anat* 102: 71–75.

Fouser L and Avner ED (1993) Normal and abnormal nephrogenesis *Am J Kidney Dis* 21: 64–70.

Inke G (1988) *The Protolobar Structure of the Human Kidney*. New York: Liss.

Lawrence WD, Whitaker D, Sugimura H, Cunha GR, Dickersin and GR Robboy SJ (1992) An ultrastructural study of the developing urogenital tract in early human fetuses. *Am J Obstet Gynecol* 167: 185–193.

Lebenthal E (Ed.) (1989) *Human Gastrointestinal Development*. New York: Raven Press.

McFadden DE and Pantzar JT (1992) Genital system. In *Developmental Pathology of the Embryo and Fetus* (Eds Dimmick JE and Kalousek DK), pp. 605–624. Philadelphia: Lippincott.

Monie IW (1989) Anatomy, embryology. In *Alimentary Tract Radiology*, 4th edn (Eds

Margoulis RA and Burhenne HJ), pp. 215–230. St. Louis: Mosby.

Satoh M (1991) Histogenesis and organogenesis of the gonad in human embryos. *J Anat* 177: 85–107.

Spitzer A, Bernstein J, Bolchis H and Edelmann CM (1991) Kidney and urinary tract. In *Neonatal-Perinatal Medicine* (Eds Faranoff AA and Martin RJ), pp. 1293–1327. St Louis: Mosby.

HEAD AND NECK

Diewert VM and Wang KY (1992) Recent advances in primary palate and midface morphogenesis research. *Critical Rev Oral Biol Med* 4: 111–130.

El-Mohandes EA, Botros KG and Bondok AA (1987) Prenatal development of the human submandibular gland. *Acta Anat* 130: 213–218.

Kjaer I (1992) Human prenatal palatal shelf elevation related to craniofacial skeletal maturation. *Eur J Orthodont* 14: 26–30.

Kramer GJ, Hoeksma JB and Prahl-Andersen B (1992) Early palatal changes in complete and incomplete cleft lip and/or palate. *Acta Anat* 144: 202–212.

Sperber GH (1989) *Craniofacial Embryology*, 4th edn London: Wright.

Sperber GH (1992) The aetiopathogenesis of craniofacial anomalies. *Ann Acad Med* 21: 708–714.

Williams ED, Toyn CE and Harach HR (1989) The ultimobranchial gland and congenital thyroid abnormalities in man. *J Path* 159: 135–141.

BRAIN

Barkovich AJ, Greesens P and Evrard P (1989) Formation, maturation, and disorders of brain neocortex. *Am J Neuroradiol* 13: 423–446.

Caviness VS (1989) Normal development of cerebral neocortex. In *Developmental Neurobiology*, vol. 12 (Eds Evrard P and Minkowski A), pp. 1–9. New York: Raven Press.

Evrard P, Kadhim HJ, de Saint-Georges P and Gadisseux J-F (1989) Abnormal development and destructive processes of the human brain during the second half of gestation. In *Developmental Neurobiology*, vol. 12 (Eds Evrard P and Minkowski A), pp. 21–41. New York: Raven Press.

Kretchmann H-J, Kammradt G, Krauthausen I, Sauer B and Lemire RJ (1988) Neural tube defects. J Am Med Assoc. 259: 558–562.

Muller F and O'Rahilly R (1991) Development of anencephaly and its variants. *Am J Anat* 190: 193–218.

Norman MG (1992) Central nervous system. In *Developmental Pathology of the Embryo and Fetus* (Eds Dimmick JE and Kalousek DK), pp. 341–382. Philadelphia: Lippincott.

Pujol R (1991) Development of the human cochlea. *Acta Otolaryngol (Stockh) Suppl 482*: 7–12.

Schatz CJ (1992) The developing brain. *Sci Am* 267: 61–67.

Williams RS (1989) Cerebral malformations arising in the first half of gestation. In *Developmental Neurobiology*, vol. 12 (Eds Evrard P and Minkowski A), pp. 11–20. Philadelphia: Lippincott.

Wingert F (1986) Brain growth in man. *Bibl Anat* 28: 1–26.

PLACENTA

Baldwin VJ (1992) Placenta. In *Developmental Pathology of the Fetus and Newborn* (Eds Dimmick JE and Kalousek DK), pp. 320–340. Philadelphia: Lippincott.

Castellucci M, Scheper M and Scheffen I (1990) The development of the human villous tree. *Anat Embryol* 181: 117–129.

Johnson M and Everitt B (1988) *Essential Reproduction*. Oxford: Blackwell.

Mayhew TM (1992) The structural basis of oxygen diffusion in the human placenta. In *Oxygen Transport in Biological Systems* (Eds Eggington S and Ross HF), pp. 79–101. Cambridge: University Press.

Index

Page numbers in bold type indicate where the main discussion can be found.
Page numbers in italic indicate where the feature is illustrated.

HUMAN EMBRYOLOGY

A clear grasp of embryology is essential to the understanding of postnatal anatomy and of congenital malformations. With this objective, **Human Embryology** provides a concise and comprehensively illustrated account of human prenatal development, for students of medicine and the allied health sciences. Recognizing the benefits of studying development in parallel with topographical as well as systems-based anatomy, material in later chapters is presented here by region (limbs, thorax, abdomen, etc), but it may equally be accessed by system using the Systems Index at the front of the book. Concise text is complemented by clear diagrams that consistently present each stage of development.

The science of embryology has its own special vocabulary; a glossary of 480 embryological terms provides essential definitions with chapter references.

M.J.T. (Turlough) FitzGerald MD PhD DSc MRIA is Professor and Chairman, Department of Anatomy, at University College, Galway, Ireland; formerly Associate Professor at the Department of Biological Structure, University of Washington School of Medicine, Seattle; and Lecturer in Anatomy at the Department of Anatomy, St Thomas's Hospital Medical School, London.

Maeve FitzGerald MB BCh BSc is Senior Lecturer, Department of Anatomy, University College, Galway, Ireland.

Cover photograph: The human fetus at about four months:
PETIT FORMAT/NESTLE/SCIENCE PHOTO LIBRARY

ISBN 0-7020-1760-4

9 780702 017605

BAILLIÈRE TINDALL, 24-28 OVAL ROAD, LONDON NW1 7DX
PRINTED IN HONG KONG